GROVANIA
A Story of Family & Faith

GROVANIA
A Story of Family & Faith

*The Lineage,
Life, and Legacy of
Dr. Samuel Brewster Leslie, Sr.*

M. Bruce Shields

White River Press
Amherst, Massachusetts

Published by White River Press
Amherst, MA 01004 • www.whiteriverpress.com

ISBNs: 978-1-935052-90-6 hardcover
           978-1-935052-87-6 paperback

Book and Cover Design by Douglas Lufkin, Lufkin Graphic Designs
Norwich, VT 05055 • www.lufkingraphics.com

All images were taken or provided by the author, and printed with the permission of the family.

Library of Congress Cataloging-in-Publication Data

Names: Shields, M. Bruce, author.
Title: Grovania : a story of family and faith / M. Bruce Shields.
Description: Amherst, Massachusetts : White River Press, 2022. | Includes
    bibliographical references.
Identifiers: LCCN 2022020190 | ISBN 9781935052876 (trade paperback)
Subjects: LCSH: Leslie, Samuel Brewster, 1874-1955. | Leslie, Samuel
    Brewster, 1874-1955--Family. | Physicians--Oklahoma--Biography. |
    Christian physicians--Oklahoma--Biography. | Christian biography--United
    States. | Okmulgee (Okla.)--Biography.
Classification: LCC R154.L46 S35 2022 | DDC 610.92 [B]--dc23/eng/20220627
LC record available at https://lccn.loc.gov/2022020190

In Loving Memory of
Blossom Eliza McKeage Leslie
A gracious and loving lady
And clearly the other half of this story

Contents

Prologue

THE OZARKS ARE AN ANCIENT RANGE of mountains that spread across much of Arkansas and Missouri and send foothills into the northeast corner of Oklahoma. They began in prehistoric times as high plateaus into which valleys were sculpted through eons of erosion, resulting in flat-topped peaks, all about the same height. With the passing of millennia, they became smooth, rolling hills, covered by dense woods that reach deep into the valleys and line the many lakes and swiftly flowing streams. The Oklahoma foothills are verdant fingers of low-lying hills amid open fields of corn, cotton, and feed grains. And, nestled amid those fields, there once stood a small, white frame church.

It was situated at the intersection of two dirt roads a few miles north of the town of Okmulgee. The building consisted of two rooms, giving it an L-shaped configuration. The entrance to the main room was through a pair of unadorned doors. A single window on either side of the entrance was of plain glass, and above the doors was perched a low steeple with a single bell that had called the faithful to worship for years. Near the intersection of the dirt roads, a low wooden sign identified the little building as "GROVANIA...A Community Church."

On a Sunday morning in the fall of 1955, a ray of sunshine had just pierced the low, gray clouds and illuminated the church, giving the windows an orange glow as if they were stained glass. There was no sign of life around the church at this early hour, but a thin cloud of dust, just up the road that led toward Okmulgee, announced the approach of a vehicle. It was a late model Buick sedan, and it slowed, turned off the road, and came to a stop on a flat surface of dirt and grass in front of the church. An elderly man stepped out from the driver's side. His thin white hair was silky and captured a glint of the morning sunlight. He wore a pale gray suit with a white shirt and a blue tie. He was tall and gaunt with slightly stooped shoulders but held himself erect and dignified as he walked gingerly around to the other side of the car. He opened the door on the passenger side and extended a hand to his companion. She looked up into his gentle hazel eyes and they shared a momentary smile. She wore a modest cotton coat over a print dress with a lace-trimmed collar that was buttoned at her neck and a long skirt that stopped just above her ankles. Her gray hair was pulled back from her creamy white face and arranged in a neat bun. She took the arm that was offered to her and the two walked slowly up to the low stone stoop and paused at the entrance. He reached into his pocket for a key, opened the door, and helped her in.

The main room had a slightly musty odor, and the air was damp and chilly. He walked over to the stove and lit a propane burner, while she distributed Bibles and hymnals, *Songs of Faith*, on the half-dozen straight wooden benches. Just then, the sound of another vehicle was heard outside. It was a vintage red pickup that had obviously seen many years of hard duty. The young family crammed into the cab were also no strangers to hard work. The man had sandy red hair that almost matched the color of his weathered face, except for the white of his upper brow where an old straw hat sat the other six days of the week. He wore a faded denim jacket over a pair of clean overalls and a white dress shirt that was slick from countless washings and ironings. His wife wore a simple gingham dress under her well-worn coat and held an infant in her arms. Beside her stood their eight-year-old daughter and their five-year-old son, who clung to his mother's skirt.

The elderly man had stepped to the front door. "Morning, Doctor Leslie," the farmer called out.

"Good morning, Tom," he replied. "Good to see you and your handsome family this lovely day."

"Shore 'nuff is a beautiful day," Tom observed.

The doctor looked up at the sky and nodded with a smile. Then he stepped back to allow the family to come inside. His smile broadened as he looked down at their son, who shyly walked over and stood beside the elderly man's leg and gazed up at him with a sense of anticipation. This brought a warm chuckle from the doctor, who bent down and picked up the little fellow and held him so he could grasp the rope and ring the bell in the church steeple, as was their custom on most Sundays.

"Good work, Luke," the doctor said. "I hear them coming." And Luke smiled from ear to ear.

As if on cue, another vehicle pulled into the parking lot. It was a station wagon with weathered wooden panels. Inside was the McIntosh family. They were members of the Creek Nation, the predominant Native American tribe in the area, although they were actually half-bloods whose kin had intermarried with Scotch-Irish descendants many generations ago. They had one teenage son still living at home, and both father and son were dressed in suit and tie.

The doctor greeted the middle-aged couple with a smile as they stepped up onto the stone stoop. "Good morning, Amos. Good morning, Miss Hettie."

"Good morning, Doc," they responded in unison, shaking his hand.

"How's that shoulder coming along, Ben?" he asked their son.

"Just about good as new, Doctor Leslie," Ben replied. "Think I can get back to throwin' the baseball pretty soon?"

"We'll see," he replied with an encouraging smile.

More cars and trucks continued to arrive, and the little church was soon filled with the chatter of friends and neighbors. Some of the men wore their best farm clothes, while others wore suits, but everyone seemed to be comfortable in each other's company. The last vehicle to arrive was an old sedan driven by an elderly African American gentleman, whose white hair suggested that he was about the same age as Dr. Leslie. He walked stooped over with the help of a cane, and the doctor came out to assist him.

"Didn't expect to see you here today, Jeremiah," he said, as he extended a helping hand.

"I's feeling a mite better this mornin', Doctuh," Jeremiah replied, leaning on the physician's arm. "Them last pills you give me seems to be helpin' some."

"Glad to hear that," the doctor replied, as the two old friends walked slowly together into the church.

The few young children in the group went with one of the ladies into the second room, which served as the Sunday School classroom, while the others took their seats on the wooden benches. A hush fell over the little congregation as Dr. Leslie stood up before them and began to speak.

"It's good to see all of you this morning. I understand Miss Lilly is still under the weather and can't be with us today, so we'll keep her in our prayers. Don't know of any others on the sick list. Glad Jeremiah is back with us after his illness," he said with a nod to the old gentleman. "So if there's no other concerns, let's bow our heads."

With all eyes closed and heads bowed, the doctor began the opening prayer.

"Father, you tell us that, where two or three are gathered in your name, there you will be, and we're grateful for your presence with us this morning. We pray that you will open our hearts and minds to receive your word in the singing of hymns, the reading of scripture, and in today's lesson, and that your word will go with us throughout the coming week. We pray this in the name of our Savior," to which all responded with a heartfelt "amen."

"Let's open our hymnals now to page 150, 'There is Power in the Blood.'" It was one of his favorites, and most of the congregation knew it by heart. They didn't have a piano or any other instrumental accompaniment, but the doctor had a passable singing voice and could usually get them off in the right key. And the gusto with which he led them and with which they responded more than compensated for any lack of musical attributes. They sang two more hymns, followed by group prayer, ending with the Lord's Prayer, and then Dr. Leslie asked one the men to read the scripture for the morning.

The reading was from the Book of Numbers, which told the story of the Israelites wandering for so many years in the desert, always with the hope of reaching the Promised Land. But when they finally came to the Jordan River with Canaan on the other side, and a reconnaissance team came back reporting "a land which floweth with milk and honey," most of the people lost their nerve. Only two of the leaders, Joshua and Caleb, voted in favor of crossing the Jordan and receiving the promised reward, saying "If the Lord delight in us, then he will bring us into this land, and give it to us." But the people could not be persuaded, and so they continued their wandering in the desert.

The reader sat down, and Dr. Leslie again stood in front of the small group. He looked down at the floor and was silent for a time, as though he was weighing his thoughts.

"This story has puzzled me for years," he began slowly, now looking up into the eyes of his listeners. "It's not surprising that many of the Israelites were afraid of what lay beyond the river. But what was it that gave people like Joshua and Caleb the courage to cross over with faith in God's promise? Why did some face that moment with fear and others with confidence?

"I suppose that, during all those years out in the desert, the people must have talked a lot among themselves about the promise they were going to receive at the end of their journey. They probably emboldened each other with a bit of bravado. But, when they finally found themselves standing at the Jordan, why did many of them lose their conviction? I can't help but think that something in the way they lived their daily lives, during all those years of wandering, must have affected how they approached that critical moment. But what was it?" He posed the question and then allowed a long pause for everyone to consider it.

"There were undoubtedly many formal religious ceremonies during those years of wandering in the Sinai," he continued. "And I can imagine many of the Israelites getting caught up in the fervor of those services, singing and praying the loudest of all and proclaiming unquestioned faith in God's promise to bring them safely to their new home. But, when they got back to their tents and their daily routine, they may have lost their fervor and allowed worldly concerns to take precedence in their lives. Other people, like Joshua and Caleb, may have maintained their fervor for God's promise through daily prayer and communion with him, which is to say they walked with God throughout each day. And maybe this lifetime relationship with God is what allowed the few to finally stand at the river with confidence in the promise of what awaited them on the other side." Again, the doctor paused, so that everyone could consider his words.

"I don't suppose we'll ever know for sure what was in the minds of those Israelites. But one thing we do know—each of us will one day stand at that river." And the people understood what he was saying.

Dr. Leslie stood silently, as though he was thinking about what he had just said and maybe wondering if he should say more. But something told him there was nothing more to say. He looked up at his friends, sitting there on the wooden benches. Some of them nodded in agreement and others bowed their heads. He looked over at his wife and thought he saw a tear in her eye. And that caused him to smile broadly in order to maintain his own composure.

"Well," he began again, with a deep sigh, "let's open our hymnals now to page 163 for the closing hymn."

The song they sang was "Shall We Gather at the River?" It was another hymn they had sung many times before, although this morning it seemed to touch them in a new way. "Soon we'll reach the shining river, Soon our pilgrimage will cease; Soon our happy hearts will quiver, With the melody of peace."

The plate was passed, Dr. Leslie gave the benediction, and then everyone got up to leave. Actually, they did not get up to leave, but to talk. This was the social time of the week for many of them, and they enjoyed catching up on the latest news and thoughts of their friends. The Leslies also enjoyed the fellowship, but on this morning they were both a bit anxious to go home. Mrs. Leslie was concerned about her husband's appearance. He looked pale and seemed to be tired. In fact, he was tired. Standing was hard on his lower back, and he was wishing that he could sit down, but did not feel they could leave until all the others had gone. So they persevered until the last truck had pulled away from the little church, and then they closed up and went to their car.

As he was opening the car door, Dr. Leslie felt a chilly breeze swirl around his head. It caused him to look up and then back toward the little white church, which held so many memories for him. And, for a moment, his thoughts seemed far away.

Once inside the car, he sat quietly for a few minutes, enjoying the silence and the relief on his back. Mrs. Leslie looked over at him with a concerned expression but said nothing. Soon he started the engine, and they pulled out onto the dirt road and headed slowly back toward Okmulgee. They rode quietly for a mile or so, both looking straight ahead, and then she broke the silence.

"Bruce, I believe that was the best lesson I ever heard you give."

He didn't respond at first but kept looking straight ahead with both hands on the steering wheel. She was not typically free with her compliments, and he knew that when they came they were from the heart and to be valued. He thought about that and about the lesson he had just given and felt that she was probably right. And he also thought, at that moment, of how blessed he was.

"Thank you, Blossom," he finally said, still looking straight ahead.

They continued to ride in silence. Maybe both of them were thinking about how blessed they were to have had the life they did together and to still have each other. But, one thing they were probably not thinking about—indeed that neither of them had any way of knowing—was that this would be their last ride together.

The following morning, Dr. Samuel Brewster Leslie suffered a major heart attack from which he would not recover. The life he had lived had prepared him well to face this moment with confidence in where he was going. But he was not ready to go. Not yet. He had lived eighty-one years and had practiced medicine in Okmulgee for fifty-three of those years and, in fact, was scheduled to see patients in his office that day. He loved life and had hoped to have a few more years to serve his patients and his family and his God. So he held on for seven weeks, and for a while it seemed that he was improving. But then, on a cold November night in 1955, he surrendered and crossed over the river.

I was fourteen years old when I stood beside my heartbroken mother in the First Methodist Church of Okmulgee to say goodbye to my grandfather. The church was overflowing with people who remembered him in many different ways—as a loving husband, a father, a grandfather—as their doctor or simply as their friend. He had maintained his membership in the Methodist Church since coming to Okmulgee, and many in the church that morning remembered him as their Sunday School teacher or as the superintendent of the Sunday School classes. Public school teachers were there who remembered him as the longtime president of the Okmulgee School Board and for his role in building so many of the schools in town. Many doctors had come to pay their respects and remembered him as a colleague and as president of the County Medical Society or as the doctor who examined them for their state license as a member of the State Board of Medical Examiners. Community leaders were there who remembered him as one of the town's leading philanthropists. And sitting in the back of the church was a small group of kindred souls who would always remember Dr. Leslie as the man who led their services in a little country church just north of town.

The life of Dr. Bruce Leslie (or S. B., as he was commonly known) is a remarkable story and is made all the more salient by the seminal times in which he lived. Born just a decade after the Civil War, he saw the country attempt to bind its wounds and join the leading nations of the free world. He saw his adopted state of Oklahoma evolve from Indian Territory to statehood and become one of the country's major contributors of energy, agriculture, and hard-working, patriotic, God-fearing people. He witnessed America survive two World Wars and the Great Depression and to emerge from it all as a dominant world power and a beacon of democracy, freedom, and hope. He saw advances in technology that had no precedent. He saw transportation evolve from the horse and buggy to the automobile and from steam engines riding the rails to airplanes sailing the skies. He saw communication evolve from the telegraph to the telephone, the radio, and television. And he saw the emergence of myriad additional wonders that electricity and other advances made possible in the modern age.

In his own profession, he witnessed the most significant advances in the history of American medicine. He saw medical education and qualifications for practicing the healing arts evolve from unregulated cottage industries in the nineteenth century to rigid standards for education and certification of doctors in the twentieth. And, with these changes, he saw the practice of medicine evolve from irrational, empirical treatments to effective therapeutic approaches based on clinical and laboratory science. When he began his practice, infectious diseases were still a worldwide scourge for which there was no reliable cure, and he lived to witness the introduction of penicillin and other antimicrobials that revolutionized medicine by providing rational treatments for civilization's greatest health threat.

And yet, through all these changing times, there was one constant in his life: an abiding faith. His simple faith in a loving Creator and Sustainer was the firm foundation that grounded him through all of life's storms and vicissitudes. It was an inheritance that he had received from the many generations that had gone before him. It came down through his ancient Scottish ancestors and remained as a guiding star for those who emigrated to Ireland and eventually to America. It went with them across the prairies of Virginia and the Carolinas, and then westward to the Ozark Mountains of Arkansas, where his grandfather established the family homestead and where he was born.

It has been well over sixty years since I stood beside my bereaved mother in that Methodist church in Okmulgee. In the interval, I have had my own medical career and am now retired, with time to tackle some unfulfilled aspirations, one of which is to tell the story of my grandfather. My hope is to convey a sense of the inspiration that his life has been to me and to so many others whose lives he touched. But I do not feel that the story would be complete if I did not tell of his ancestry and of the remarkable times in which he lived, all of which shaped the person he was. So the initial chapters trace the history of the Leslie clan from the ancient Scots through generations of migration in Ireland and America to his birth in the Ozark Mountains.

The historical basis for the story is derived from many sources, most of which are listed in the References and Acknowledgements. But this only provides a skeleton of the story, without much of the feeling for how it might have been. In the hope of adding this element to the story—of putting a little flesh on the bones—I have been rather liberal with poetic license. While the basic facts are accurate (to the best of my knowledge), I have allowed my imagination to run free—surmising how it might have been to have lived in those times. So although many of the vignettes are fictional, I believe that the values and feelings that I have added to augment the facts are representative of those who lived the story.

This then is the account of one family and the times in which they lived. But it could be the story of so many families whose ancestors came to America in search of a better life. It is the American story. Maybe it will remind you of someone in your own family who inspired you. And, for all of us, it may recall the countless people in our American heritage who persevered through the challenges and heartaches of creating a new way of living, that we might all enjoy a richer life.

PART ONE

Lineage and Early Years

CHAPTER 1

Scotland
c. 1069

BARTOFF RESTED IN HIS SADDLE and gazed for the first time out across a vast panorama of austere and awesome landscape.

Unable to sleep on such a momentous day, he had risen well before dawn. He quietly saddled his horse and rode slowly over the courtyard cobblestones, trying not to disturb the pigs and chickens and the people asleep inside. As he rode out into the bleak predawn darkness, he saw the barren moor ascend gradually on either side of the rocky road until it faded from view in the moonless darkness. He had been warned to be on the alert for inhospitable locals, who were known to take advantage of lone travelers. But nothing was visible in any direction, and he seemed to have the entire bleak countryside to himself.

In the silence and solitude, his thoughts drifted back over the remarkable events that had led to this moment. He contemplated once again how the winds of fortune blow so suddenly and unexpectedly into our lives, and with such force. He marveled at how abruptly they may alter one's course in life, sending us in directions we could never have anticipated. And he smiled to think that even the storms that seem to be the darkest may guide us into safe harbors with unexpected blessings for ourselves and our generations to come. But most of all he thought about Margaret.

He had met her in Hungary, where Margaret was born during her father's exile from England. She was only a child when they first met and, although he was a few years older, they became inseparable friends. They seemed to share all the same joys in life—a love of nature, of the open glens and wooded dells and all the creatures that live there. They loved to wade through streams and climb trees and run through grassy meadows. They loved to watch the clouds drift by in the day and count the stars at night and wonder at the mystery of it all. As they grew older, both developed a passion for horseback riding, although it was Bartoff who would become the expert horseman. He had the physique for it—tall, with strong but slightly stooped shoulders and wide hips with muscular thighs—and he cut a handsome figure atop any steed. Margaret would often ride behind him on a special saddle, and when they forded a flowing stream, she would laugh when he invariably admonished her, "Grip fast."

The two young people also shared a strong faith. Margaret was especially known for her piousness and spent hours in prayer and in the reading of her Bible. Although Bartoff was more inclined to find his spiritual inspiration in nature, he admired Margaret for what he called her saintliness and often knelt beside her to pray in their chapel. There came a time when he realized that he loved Margaret and rather suspected that she felt the same way about him. But she was a princess of the English royal family and, although he was considered a nobleman, the difference in their status was such that their love could never be more than that of a brother and sister. And that was enough for him—as long as they could be together and he could protect her.

Her father brought his family back to England when Princess Margaret was about ten years old, but he died shortly thereafter and she grew up with her brother, Prince Edgar. Bartoff came with them from Hungary and held a special position in their court as keeper of the horses and unofficial protector of the princess. Those were turbulent times for England. As Margaret was approaching her twentieth year, the Norman invaders under William the Conqueror brought an end to 600 years of Anglo-Saxon rule at the Battle of Hastings in 1066. William treated Margaret's family well until her brother made the fatal mistake of supporting an abortive rebellion in northern England. Edgar and his family attempted an escape back to Hungary, but their ship was blown off course toward Scotland, and they found safe harbor in a small inlet off the coast of Fife, where friendly inhabitants gave them shelter. And so it was that Bartoff was venturing into the Scottish countryside that dark morning, with a sense of apprehension for what the day might hold.

Returning from his reverie, he realized that the world about him had been changing. Heavy gray clouds could now be seen hanging low overhead, allowing faint rays of early dawn light to filter through and illuminate the vast landscape in pale blue hues. Having reached the highest point of his journey, he paused to take in the scene that stretched before him. Verdant grasslands swept down gently amid massive outcroppings of gray stone, thickets of low, dark green trees, and swaths of faint purples and yellows that clung close to the ground. Far below, the terrain leveled off and spread out in undulating patterns of hills and dells until they disappeared into the distant morning mist. Off to one side, a narrow shaft of sunlight found passage through the heavy clouds and illuminated the ridges with an almost iridescent green, while long, dark shadows stretched through the intervening valleys. The light sparkled off the slate gray waters of distant lochs and danced on the tortuous streams that bubbled over rocky beds and meandered around groves of trees and shrubs. An arched stone bridge crossed a stream at one point, and a few farmhouses, with their light-colored walls and dark, thatched roofs, punctuated the otherwise empty countryside, while small white dots of sheep grazed nearby.

The vastness and loneliness of the scene that spread before him sent a foreboding chill through Bartoff's bones. And yet, at the same time, he felt a sense of exhilaration to realize that somewhere out there in this strange new world might lie his future. With a profound feeling of gratitude, he closed his eyes and said a prayer of thanksgiving. He gave thanks for the winds that had guided them to this place and for the safety and good health that they had been granted. And he said a special prayer for Margaret, whose life he sensed was about to undergo a most propitious change.

Just then, a gentle breeze brushed across his face, prompting Bartoff to open his eyes and squint into the intensifying light of the day. He noticed that the wind was picking up, blowing away the distant mist and revealing something on the far horizon that he had not seen earlier—an approaching army. He judged there to be some fifty horsemen coming over the farthest ridge. And, as he squinted to see more clearly, he realized that the number was growing as more riders ascended the ridge and advanced in his direction. In all, he concluded there must be several hundred. As he continued his observation, he could see that some of the horsemen in the lead were holding flags that whipped in the wind. Although he could not make out the colors of the flags, he felt rather certain that he knew whom they represented: Malcolm III—King of Scotland.

Indeed, it was King Malcolm, leading his men down the slopes and onto the moor in the direction of Bartoff's position. Behind him, the flags of his kingdom fluttered from a half dozen poles that were held aloft by his standard bearers. The noblemen of his court spread out behind the flags, followed by the officers and soldiers of Malcolm's private guard. Finally, a host of servants struggled to keep up, their carts and animals laden with provisions and supplies.

The Scotland that Malcolm had inherited was still in a nascent and unsettled state, having been united by his great-grandfather, Malcolm II, only a half century earlier. For more than a thousand years, it had been a land of fiercely independent clans, mostly of Celtic origin. The inhabitants eventually formed into four races, of which the Picts were the largest. They ruled for most of that period, until they were conquered by a warlike race from Northern Ireland called the Scots. In the ninth century, Kenneth MacAlpin succeeded in establishing a monarchy over most of the land, which became known as Scotland. However, it was not until early in the eleventh century that Malcolm II, a descendant of MacAlpin, brought the final race, the Anglo-Saxon Lothians, under Scottish rule. He was succeeded by his grandson, Duncan, who was killed in battle by Macbeth. After a seventeen-year reign, Macbeth was killed by Duncan's elder son, Malcolm III, who ascended to the throne in 1058, beginning his thirty-five-year rule.

Malcolm had good reason to feel sanguine about the future of his kingdom as he galloped slowly across the moor that morning. The first ten years of his reign had seen significant advances in Scotland, with progress toward a more modern state. He had become known as Malcolm Canmore, from the Gaelic *ceann mòr,* meaning "Great Chief," attesting to the respect that he enjoyed among his subjects. But there was one thing he lacked—an heir, or more precisely, a wife to give him a son. He was in his fortieth year, a widower, and by far the country's most eligible bachelor. From age nine until he returned to Scotland as king, he had lived in England, where he was acquainted with Prince Edgar and his sister, Princess Margaret, who was then still a child and somewhat of a tomboy, albeit with an esteemed reputation. When he learned that the royal family had unexpectedly come to Scotland and was not far from his castle in Dunfermline, he sent an envoy to arrange a meeting. And so it was that Malcolm was leading his men across the heath in the early morning hours toward the position where a lone rider was observing them.

Bartoff remained motionless, his eyes keenly fixed on the approaching army until he felt certain about their identity. Then he gave a sharp jerk to the reins of his horse and headed back down the rock-strewn path from which he had just come. He had been riding some distance when he saw a small party of riders coming up over a far distant rise. Knowing that they would be anxious to hear the news, he spurred his horse to a gallop and was soon pulling up beside his companions, who were indeed in a sense of silent anticipation. The riders were led by Edgar and Margaret, followed by a half dozen noblemen from their court. No words were spoken, but all eyes were on Bartoff, who knew they were awaiting his report.

"He comes," Bartoff announced with his typical conservation of words.

Edgar acknowledged the report with a grim nod, obviously concerned as to the true motives of the Scotsmen, who had not always been particularly friendly with the English. Bartoff turned his gaze toward Margaret and thought that she had never looked lovelier, despite the worried countenance that she could not hide. He gave her a wink, which she returned with her best attempt at a brave smile. Then Edgar gave the signal for the party to proceed, and they continued their slow, tedious trek over the rough, unforgiving land.

By the time they returned to the peak from which Bartoff had made his observation, he was met with a most unexpected sight. Malcolm's party had stopped in the valley below and appeared to be setting up a small village in the open countryside. There was a large white tent with flags fluttering from all corners, behind which stood several smaller tents. Smoke rose from fires near the small tents, and a large number of people seemed to be moving purposefully in all directions. As the little party was taking in this curious scene, a rider came galloping toward them bearing the king's standard. He brought his horse to a halt about fifty feet from them, dismounted and walked up to within comfortable speaking distance.

"His Majesty, Malcolm Canmore, King of Scotland, bids ye warm greetings and welcome to his kingdom," the messenger began, with a low, formal bow toward Edgar and Margaret. "And he requests the honor of thine presence this day in his tent."

"Tell the king that his humble servants are most grateful for His Majesty's generosity," Edgar responded with equal formality and gravity, "and that it be our honor to accept his most gracious invitation."

With that, the messenger bowed again, returned to his horse and galloped back to convey Edgar's reply, while the English party proceeded slowly down the grassy slope toward the encampment. As they approached the king's tent, three men of noble bearing walked out to greet them. They indicated that Edgar and Margaret were to come with them, while the members of their court could join the Scottish noblemen for rest and refreshment.

For a structure that had been erected so hastily, the interior of the king's tent had a remarkably stately ambience, with a thick red carpet covering the entire floor and exquisite tapestries gracing the walls. At the far end of the tent were three chairs of heavy polished oak with rich inlays of gold and jewels. From the middle chair, King Malcolm rose with a graceful, regal bearing and stepped forward to greet his guests. He had changed from his riding clothes into his finest kingly raiment and, although he would not have wanted his guests to know it, had spent a bit more time than usual on his appearance. And the effort achieved its goal. He had a ruggedly handsome, chiseled face, with a short, meticulously trimmed beard and wavy auburn hair on which was set a simple gold crown. He was of average height, with a better than average physique, and he comported himself with an air in keeping with his royal stature. However, he momentarily lost his kingly bearing when his eyes fell on Margaret. It had been more than a decade since he had last seen her, during which time she had grown from a gangling child to a beautiful young woman. The fact that she did not have the benefit of changing from her riding clothes seemed to only make her all the more fetching. Her long, flaxen, slightly windblown hair caressed her delicate shoulders, and the same wind had given her cheeks a natural blush that no cosmetic could have matched. But the most striking feature was her soft, pale blue eyes, which spoke of wisdom and gentleness as they met Malcolm's. The king was fatally smitten on the spot.

The three enjoyed a long, cordial visit, as the winds of Scottish history blew about their tent. Eventually, they emerged and proceeded to introduce the noblemen of their respective courts. When Margaret came to Bartoff, she introduced him as her "dearest friend." This caused Bartoff to blush and Malcolm to feel a momentary sense of jealousy. But the king's feelings were quickly assuaged as he looked into the hazel eyes of Margaret's friend and saw humility and sincerity. Here was a man he could trust.

"Any friend of Princess Margaret shall surely be a friend of mine," he said to Bartoff, who again blushed and bowed long and low.

That afternoon, a feast was spread out on a long table in front of the king's tent around which the noblemen sat, with Malcolm at the head and Edgar and Margaret on either side. Bartoff, positioned near the opposite end of the table, kept a close eye on Margaret and her host. It was not lost on him that Malcolm could not seem to take his eyes off the princess and treated her as though they were the only two at the table. Now it was Bartoff who felt a twinge of jealousy. He had known this day would come and yet, as much as he had tried to prepare himself for it, he found himself struggling with his emotions. But his greatest concern had always been for Margaret's welfare, and he felt rather certain that the winds were continuing to blow her life on a most favorable course. What he could not have known at that moment, however, was that the new direction in Margaret's life would alter not only the course of Scottish history but also the future of his own lineage.

Bartoff's intuition was quite prescient. Three months after their meeting on the moor, Malcolm and Margaret were married in Dunfermline. Again Bartoff had to struggle with his emotions as he stood among the noblemen and ladies of honor, watching his best friend—looking more radiant than ever—come gracefully down the long aisle to where Malcolm waited for her. But his emotions were mixed by a sense of both loss and gain, as he reminded himself that Margaret was marrying a good man who offered her a bright future, and that he too stood to benefit from this royal matrimony.

During the brief courtship, Bartoff gradually gained the confidence and respect, if not the affection, of the king, who began to see him as a trusted member of his inner circle. The king's opinion of Bartoff was a consequence not only of the young man's sincere demeanor and his devotion to Margaret, but also of the fact that he shared the king's passion for horses and was an excellent horseman. Shortly after the wedding, Bartoff was appointed Lord Chamberlain to Queen Margaret and was given the honor and duty of carrying the Queen on his horse. Like old times, she would laugh each time their horse galloped across a flowing stream and he would admonish her, "Grip fast."

Almost from the beginning, the influence of Queen Margaret was felt in the Scottish royal court and throughout the kingdom. She was not only a saintly woman, but also a very determined one, and she soon brought an element of culture and a more civilized nature to Malcolm's court. Because of his English education, the king was inclined to grant the majority of his queen's wishes, even to the extent of moving the cultural center of his kingdom southward into Anglo-Saxon Lothian, at the risk of seriously offending his Celtic subjects in the northern highlands. Margaret also took the Scottish clergy in hand, which proved to be a greater challenge, owing to the passion with which the people held their religious beliefs.

During the middle of the sixth century, Christian missionaries from Ireland began coming to Scotland, and by the seventh century all four of the ancient races had converted to Christianity. However, the practices of the Celtic Church differed considerably from those in England, not to mention Rome, and the Scottish clergy were quite dismayed when Margaret sought to impose the English religious practices of celibacy, poverty, and the like on them. Conflict between the Celtic Church and the wealthier, more organized Roman Church had been going on for some time. The Celts eventually yielded, although they would always contend that the Celtic Church gave love, while the Roman Church gave law. And Margaret's influence on the Church of Scotland sought to ensure that it would have both.

Bartoff watched Margaret's ascendancy and success in the Scottish court with a sense of detached amusement. He could have warned their new countrymen that they were wasting their time in trying to dissuade her from a goal once her mind was set. She had always been able to get her way—including with him—through a combination of beguiling charm and stubborn determination. As for Bartoff, he was interested neither in affairs of state nor in becoming embroiled in contentious matters of any sort. He was more than content to look after Margaret and take care of their horses, and this further increased his favor in the eyes of the king, who soon appointed him as overseer of all the royal horses. But his equine responsibilities were not the only interest that had begun to occupy Bartoff's attention in Malcolm Canmore's court.

The Queen had a small group of well-bred young women, known as "ladies of honor," who served various functions in the royal court. This was one of the traditions that Margaret had encouraged as a result of her English upbringing, and she was diligent to ensure not only that each lady was from the finest of noble clans, but also that they shared her values of piety and virtue. Among these ladies of honor was one who everyone agreed stood out from all the others in the extent to which she exemplified the Queen's values. Her name was Marianne. Physically, she bore a remarkable resemblance to Margaret, with long flaxen hair, pale blue eyes, and a petite figure. But in demeanor, she was quite different, with a demure, reserved personality and a modesty that caused her to blush whenever she became the subject of attention. And for some time now she had been the subject of a certain young man's attention.

Margaret had observed the way that Bartoff looked at Marianne, who she suspected also had a special interest in the handsome horseman. She decided that they were well suited for each other but knew that Bartoff was as shy as Marianne and feared that the two would never do more than admire each other from afar unless she stepped in. And so she began to arrange social functions that would bring them into closer contact. Subtlety not being one of Margaret's strengths, the two young people quickly saw through her trickery, although neither had any objections. In fact, they were quite grateful for the Queen's intervention, as they began spending more and more time together, and it soon became obvious to all that their feelings for each other were more than just casual. Months passed, however, and the first anniversary of their courtship was approaching without Bartoff showing any sign of taking action toward matrimony.

Both Marianne and Margaret were perplexed and were beginning to despair of Bartoff's inaction, when they met one day to analyze the situation. Marianne, with a painful shyness, assured the Queen of her love for Bartoff and allowed that she was quite sure he felt the same toward her, but was puzzled by his apparent lack of interest in marriage. Margaret, knowing Bartoff better than anyone, felt that it was more than just a matter of shyness on his part and promised Marianne that she would do what she could. That evening, she discussed the matter with Malcolm, who had, over time, developed a special affection for Bartoff and agreed that Marianne would be the perfect wife for him. He told Margaret to leave the matter to him.

In addition to their common passion for horses, Malcolm and Bartoff shared another rather unusual interest—they were both fond of poetry and enjoyed amusing each other by speaking in verse. Shortly after the royal couple had their discussion, Bartoff was summoned to an audience with the king, where it was obvious from the twinkle in Malcolm's eyes that he was about to be regaled with the latest royal poetry.

"Providence brought thee from the sea; a noble Scotsman now ye be," Malcolm quoted with a mix of humor and sincerity.

Bartoff smiled and blushed and bowed his head in acknowledgement of the compliment, although he felt quite sure that he had not been called into the king's presence to be congratulated on his assimilation into the Scottish race.

"Time 'tis nigh that thou shouldst plan," Malcolm continued, "thy estate to build and raise a clan."

"*So that's what it's all about*," Bartoff thought, with an inward chuckle. He had no doubt that Margaret was behind it, but he decided to play along with the rhyming game.

"But where, O' King, dare I begin; a clan to raise with na' kith nor kin?"

Now it was Malcolm who was chuckling, as he realized that neither man was doing a very good job of concealing their true intentions from the other. But he also suspected that Bartoff was becoming a bit uncomfortable with the direction of the conversation and felt it was time to drop the rhymes and be more direct.

"Hast thou not, my friend, found any among our fair lasses with whom ye might see eternity?"

"Aye, I have, your Highness."

"And who might she be?" Malcolm pried with that twinkle in his eye.

"The Lady Marianne, my Lord," Bartoff responded, with a painful blush, strongly suspecting that the king already knew the answer before he announced it.

"Ah, yes. A most agreeable lass. Ye have chosen well, my friend," Malcolm exclaimed with a broad, satisfied smile. "And I have it on the best authority that the young lady reciprocates thy feelings." Then he paused, and his countenance changed to one of a more serious, fatherly nature. "But, if ye will permit me to ask, what causes thee to delay in asking for the fair lass's hand? I can assure ye that the Queen and I are most anxious to grant these nuptials, and with our most heartfelt blessings."

There was a long, awkward silence. It was obvious that Bartoff was struggling with his emotions, as he considered how to respond.

"O' King, thou hast been most fair to me," he began slowly and pensively, "and words ca' nay express my gratitude. But, despite thy generosity, I am but a humble servant, with na' wealth nor land to offer one who would be my bride."

Malcolm let out a long sigh of relief and almost laughed at the alleviation he felt from Bartoff's explanation. But he could see that this was anything but a laughing matter for his young friend, and he maintained his paternal demeanor as he proceeded to relate his true reason for summoning Bartoff—a revelation that nearly knocked the horseman off his feet and would dramatically alter the course of his life and that of all his lineage to come.

"Bartoff, my friend, thou hast been a loyal and trustworthy servant since the day that Providence brought us together," the king began with a slow and thoughtful choice of words, "and 'tis men like thee that I must have in my kingdom, not only now but for generations to come. And so I wish to grant thee land in Scotland wherein thou canst build thy estate and raise thy clan."

Malcolm paused to allow this startling proclamation to sink in with Bartoff, who was totally lost for words. The king then went on to explain the process by which this granted land would be delineated. He told him the direction in which he should ride his horse, which was toward the moor where they had first met, and roughly the land that he could claim, but he could not resist one last whimsical verse.

"The point where thou must rest thy steed, will mark the land to thee I deed."

Bartoff was stunned and now completely incapable of speech. Seeing his emotion, the king rose to indicate that the audience was over. Bartoff also rose quickly, but then dropped to his knee and kissed the outstretched hand of his sovereign, as tears moistened his hazel eyes.

Bartoff was now faced with two tasks, the first of which he feared far more than the second. On a moonlit evening, which he was quite sure Margaret had arranged, he met with Marianne and awkwardly asked her if she would consent to be his wife. Marianne's first thought was to wonder how in the world the royal couple had pulled it off, but that didn't really matter at this most important moment in her life. She was overcome with a profound sense of thankfulness and said a silent prayer as she brushed back tears from her eyes and nodded her head.

The second task was actually a relief, as he saddled his horse to ride out of Dunfermline and back toward the moors of Fife. It was not that he took any pleasure in being away from Marianne—to the contrary, he felt a true sense of melancholy to be leaving her for even a short while. But the excitement at court surrounding the announcement of the forthcoming wedding caused him considerable embarrassment, and he never seemed to know quite what to say when someone congratulated him. So he was more than content to leave the planning of the wedding to Marianne and Margaret as he rode off to find the land for their new home.

Riding along in the early hours of the day, his mind drifted back to that first fateful morning when life had forever changed for both Margaret and himself. He marveled for the umpteenth time at how the winds of fortune blow providentially through our lives, and he said another brief prayer of gratitude. Soon he was noticing landmarks that had once seemed foreign, but now were beginning to have the feel of home—the arched stone bridge over a meandering brook, the thatched homes with sheep in the nearby fields, the patches of purple and yellow, which he had learned to call heather and whin, and always the grassy slopes of the glens and dells. It was a beautiful day, and the hours passed with neither horse nor rider recognizing that fatigue was setting in. Eventually, however, they came to a large stone, which Bartoff felt was a suitable lesse.

The term lesse, as Bartoff had come to understand it, referred to a stone that was used to demarcate property held under lease, or by the lessee. He paused for a moment and considered making this the limit of the land that he would claim for his grant. But his horse did not seem ready to rest quite yet, and so they continued on a bit further. Eventually they came to a place called Garish, and it was here that the horse gave out and they rested for the night. As Bartoff lay on his blanket beneath the twinkling stars, with his horse tied to a nearby tree, he let his mind play as he gazed across the moor and envisioned a home—maybe even a modest castle—with lights shining in the windows, a loving wife inside overseeing the evening meal, and children playing merrily about. He had never felt such contentment. He closed his eyes and said a prayer of sincere thankfulness as he drifted off into a most peaceful sleep.

Upon his return to Dunfermline, Bartoff was again summoned before the king, this time to make his report, which he presented in rhyme.

"Between a lesse ley and a mair [more], my horse was tired and I stopped there."

Malcolm laughed heartily and then thought for a moment, especially about the "lesse ley" phrase, and then with the twinkle in his eye, he responded with his own verse.

"Lord Leslie shalt thou be, and thy heirs after thee."

And so it was that Bartoff became known as Bartoff of Leslie.

The wedding, of course, was not nearly as grand as that for Malcolm and Margaret, but for two young people, it could not have been grander. Bartoff and Marianne wasted no time in planning and working toward the establishment of their own clan. Together they designed their home, which soon began to rise as a modest stone house on a grassy slope not far from the spot where Bartoff and his horse had rested that first night near the meandering brook and in sight of the arched bridge. The young couple worked hard to make their house a home and to improve the land about it with gardens and fields for their crops and pastures for their sheep. Before long, the children that Bartoff had once dreamed of were running through the house and about the fields. They named their first child Malcolm and were blessed with a large family of healthy children. Over time, they added rooms to their home as their family expanded, and the dream that Bartoff had envisioned on that night under the stars finally became a reality.

King Malcolm and Queen Margaret were also blessed with a large family, and life seemed good in the kingdom of Malcolm Canmore— in large measure due to Margaret's influence. But peace always seemed to be a short-lived respite in their lives, and the threat of war forever hung over the land like a dark, menacing cloud.

For a thousand years, the inhabitants of the southern British Isle, first under the occupation of the Romans, then the Anglo-Saxons, and now the Normans, had challenged the northern races for the boundaries that divided their lands. Scotland now enjoyed a fragile truce with England under the rule of William I, also known as William the Conqueror, but there was still no agreement as to the demarcations that separated their two countries. Malcolm believed that the northern counties of England, Northumberland and Cumberland, rightfully belonged to Scotland, and he was committed to returning them to his kingdom, even if it meant war. He called his noblemen together in a council to seek their advice, but more precisely to receive their endorsement to go to war with England.

Bartoff had held a strong opinion on the matter for some time and was dismayed to find himself on the side of the small minority in the king's council. He had never been comfortable with any form of confrontation, whether verbal or physical, and he was especially opposed to war without profound provocation. It was not that he was an unqualified pacifist—he would not hesitate to take up arms to protect Marianne and their children or his king and queen—but he felt that war should be a last resort, when one's life and freedom could not otherwise be assured. In particular, he could not rationalize the concept that acquisition of more land was worth the loss of human life. "What amount of land is equal to one human life?" he asked the king and his council, but his rhetorical question fell on deaf ears, as the vast majority counseled that it was their sovereign right to expand their kingdom. Bartoff was especially disappointed when Malcolm accepted the majority opinion of the council and prepared his army to march south. But, despite his strong opposition to the conquest, Bartoff remained loyal to his monarch and, having done all he could to prevent it, he now helped his country prepare for war.

In the year 1070, Malcolm's forces were successful in capturing the two northern English counties, but William retaliated two years later by marching north with his Norman army and defeating the Scots, forcing King Malcolm to pay homage. Because the Scottish King was still popular in the English court, however, the two countries maintained their fragile but amicable relationship over the course of the next two decades. Those were trying years for Margaret, who was always suspicious of Malcolm's Norman "friends" and continually feared for her husband's life. She spent more and more time in the chapel, praying for God's mercy, which added further to her reputation of saintliness. And then, in 1093, her greatest fear was realized when Malcolm was ambushed and killed by a Norman soldier, whom he had considered his friend. When Queen Margaret received the news, she remained in the chapel, where she died three days after the loss of her husband.

Bartoff and Marianne were inconsolable in the loss of their two dearest friends within such a short period of time. Of even greater concern for Bartoff and his sons, who were now among the influential leaders in Scotland, was the turmoil in which their country struggled under a succession of weak, insecure kings. But in 1124, David, the ninth son of Malcolm , assumed the throne of Scotland as King David I. He had received a Norman education in England, and Bartoff could see in him the same virtues that his father had possessed. He ruled for the next thirty years, largely replacing the Celtic way of life with an Anglo-Norman order and bringing many reforms of justice and sound administration to Scotland. In memory of his saintly mother, David had a tiny, simple building constructed at the summit of the citadel of Edinburgh Castle, called St. Margaret's Chapel.

Bartoff did not live to see the coronation of David I, having died three years earlier. But the clan that he and Marianne established would expand exponentially over the generations to come, providing many distinguished leaders of Scottish history. Their son Malcolm was knighted by King William the Lion and was granted additional land in Aberdeenshire. Malcolm's oldest son, Norman, received still further land grants and was appointed constable of Invenrie. He was killed in the Crusades, but successive generations held his office of constable. By the fourteenth century, surnames were starting to be used, and another Norman, the fifth generation to hold the Leslie title, became known as Norman Leslie. He was knighted, served in the Parliament of King Robert Bruce, and held the office of deputy chamberlain of Scotland.

In the centuries that followed, the Leslie clan continued to occupy important roles in the annals of Scotland. Some made the history books, such as John Leslie, the sixteenth century historian and bishop of Ross who was envoy to Mary Queen of Scots. Others became prominent military leaders, which undoubtedly would not have pleased Bartoff. But the vast majority of Leslies simply lived out their lives as common citizens of Scotland, making their contributions where they could. Many would eventually leave the country for various reasons, finding their destiny in far-flung corners of the world—wherever the winds of fortune might blow.

But there is a motto on the Leslie Coat of Arms that will forever recall the first Leslie and two young people riding joyfully together on a galloping horse across flowing Scottish streams—"Grip Fast."

CHAPTER 2

Ireland

c. 1680

J OHN LESLIE STOOD ON THE AFTERDECK and gazed through pensive hazel eyes at the misty blue outline of Scotland as it gradually faded into the distant horizon. His tall, lanky frame was stooped a bit more than usual from the burden that weighed on his heart. With one bony hand, he gripped tightly to the rail of the ship, as it heaved to the wind and lurched over the white, foaming waves. In his other hand, he held a Bible. Of the scant possessions he had brought with him, none was more cherished. The Bible was his connection to the past and his hope for the future. But it had not always been that way.

His mother had bought the Bible for him soon after he learned to read. It was a leather-bound copy of the recently published King James Version, with gold edging and a metal latch. He proudly wrote his name on the first page along with the date, which he would always remember as a most propitious day in his life. On the day he received his Bible, he began a daily schedule of reading. At his mother's suggestion, he started at the beginning—Genesis—"In the beginning, God created...." He was fascinated by the story of creation and found inspiration in many passages, especially in Proverbs and Psalms. But questions began to arise in his mind as he got into the parts about wars and the deviousness of people and what seemed to his youthful reasoning as God's approval and even promotion of their warlike behavior. Is this what religion was all about? Didn't the Bible say "Thou shalt not kill," and hadn't he been taught in church to "Love thy neighbor as thyself"? At the same time that he was trying to reconcile these teachings against the stories of violence that he found in his Bible, he was becoming increasingly disturbed by the never-ending contention among his countrymen. And two things made this strife seem even worse to the young John Leslie: that much of the underlying source of discord seemed to be differences in religious beliefs and that among the leaders of the fighting were relatives within his own clan.

King James had ruled over both Scotland and England and was succeeded by his son, Charles I, who made the fatal mistake of attempting to align the Presbyterian Church of Scotland with the Anglican Church of England. When he tried to impose a "Book of Common Prayer" on the Scots, it was more than they could take. It led to the Scottish revolt. And the leader of the Scottish forces was Alexander Leslie, also known in John's clan as old Uncle Sandy.

John Leslie was born in 1640, the same year that Uncle Sandy and the Scots defeated Charles's English army. In an attempt to make amends with his Scottish subjects, Charles freely bestowed honors and peerages, including naming Alexander Leslie the Earl of Leven. But John's family did not fare as well. His father was killed in the battle, leaving his mother to raise her only child.

Matters continued to go poorly for Charles I. The English Parliament turned against him, and the Scots joined the Parliamentarian army in exchange for the guaranteed preservation of their reform religion. Old Sandy was joined by another clansman, his nephew David Leslie, who led the Scottish cavalry. Under the leadership of the two Leslies, Charles's Royalist army was defeated, and Charles surrendered to the Scots, who turned him over to the English Parliament. Oliver Cromwell, a member of Parliament, arose as the new leader of the land and became a virtual dictator for the next thirteen years.

John was nine when news came that Cromwell had put Charles on trial and had him beheaded. Even though the Scots registered strong opposition to the execution of the former king, this was the final blow for the young Leslie. He had been losing faith in all forms of government and was becoming increasingly disillusioned with religion, which seemed to be the government's justification for all their heinous acts. The day finally came when John closed his Bible with no thought of ever opening it again, and told his mother that he no longer cared to attend church, which he now saw as hypocritical.

The Cromwell years were tumultuous for Scotland and for the Leslie clan. The radical faction of the Scottish government now ruled Scotland and wanted to bring back the monarchy. Charles I had left behind an heir, the Prince of Wales, whom the Scottish Parliament proceeded to crown King Charles II. This was tantamount to declaring war on England. Cromwell's army attacked the Scots, who were now under the command of General David Leslie. Things did not go as well for Scotland this time. Receiving ill-advised orders from Charles and the Scottish religious commissars, the Scots were defeated at the Battle of Worcester in 1651. Leslie and his men escaped to the north, and Charles went into exile in Europe until the death of Cromwell, after which he returned as Charles II of England. And this is when things went from bad to worse for Scotland.

Charles sought revenge on the Scots, who he felt had opposed him. He restored an Episcopal order of worship, which the Scottish people refused to accept, and the Scots staged a rebellion that was brutally crushed by Charles's forces.

John could recall those terrible days as though they were yesterday. By that time in his life, however, he was beginning to find answers to the conflicting thoughts that tortured his mind—the senseless killings and brutality that people rationalized in the name of religion. When he had closed his Bible, several years earlier, and told his mother that he no longer wished to attend church, she did not attempt to dissuade him. But in her heart she agonized for the soul of her son. One day, as she was cleaning his room, she noticed that the bookmark in his Bible was in the last few books of the Old Testament, which gave her a thought. At dinner that night, she asked John if he had read any of the New Testament in his Bible. He explained that he had taken her advice and started at the beginning and had not finished the Old Testament before making the decision to stop reading. She allowed a few minutes of silence, as they both continued to eat, and then suggested that he might be surprised by what he would find in the New Testament.

John had been hardened by years of cynicism and was inclined to dismiss his mother's comment, and his Bible remained untouched for another week. But he loved and respected his mother, and largely out of deference to her he picked it up one evening and opened it to the first chapter of Matthew. It was a slow start, with a genealogy and the story of Jesus's birth, the latter of which he already knew. But, as he got further into the book, something began to impress and then amaze him: there was no mention of war or of taking revenge against one's enemies. Instead it talked about healing the sick and comforting the downtrodden and even loving your enemies. "Well, that is certainly a different way," he thought. But he had heard it before and had failed to see its application in the world around him. Then one day, as he continued to read, he had an epiphany—he discovered that Jesus had felt the same way as he did about the hypocrites, who on the outside appear to people as righteous but on the inside are full of hypocrisy and wickedness. He read and reread every book in the New Testament several times and gradually came to believe that the true nature of God was not to be found in the actions of men—their wars and their hatred—but in the life and teachings of Jesus—his love and his compassion. This was the turning point in John's life. He now felt strongly that, no matter what people around him might say or do, even in the name of religion, there would always be an anchor to keep him grounded in the truth. And yet he would need that faith in spades to cope with the atrocities that were yet to come.

Charles II never returned to Scotland but appointed his brother James, Duke of York, to govern it as the king's viceroy. James, a Catholic, tried to restore Catholic worship in Edinburgh. But the main problem in Scotland remained the attempt to reconcile the Presbyterians with the Episcopal order of church government. James added to the fury by ordering Scots to swear an oath of loyalty to the king, all of which led to uprisings that were brutally suppressed in an era that became known as "the Killing Time." Thousands died during those awful years, and many tried to escape to wherever they could find refuge. Some went to the Ulster Plantation of Northern Ireland, which had been created early in the century as a place where Scotsmen of means could settle in order to promote the Protestant faith. Not surprisingly, this led to tension with the Catholics, although an uneasy peace existed in Ireland at the moment that John Leslie was approaching its shores.

At first it was not possible to tell if what he saw was truly land or just the trick that the ocean's horizon can play on the eyes. John kept his vision focused on the distant point where sky met water—or maybe land. He had moved to the front of the ship, where many other passengers now stood along the railing in eager anticipation of the first sighting of Ireland.

A myriad of thoughts went through John's mind as he stood there with the other passengers. He thought about his mother and how thankful he was that he had begun taking her to church again while she was still able. And he was thankful that she had died peacefully before having to witness the worst of the Killing Time. Leaving Scotland had been like tearing his heart out. But, with his mother gone and the constant dangers at home, especially for those who bore the name Leslie, it made no sense to stay.

The passengers now were shouting that land had been sighted, and John looked up to gaze for the first time upon the coastline of Ireland—his new home. He bowed his head, closed his eyes, said a prayer, and gripped his Bible tightly.

Arthur McIntosh kept a close eye on the tall, lanky stranger who had just entered his store. Decades of unrest had taught him to be suspicious of nearly everyone, especially ones he did not recognize.

McIntosh was a third-generation immigrant to Ireland, his grandparents having come over from Scotland early in the seventeenth century with the first wave of the Ulster Plantation. They had not exactly been greeted with open arms, since the Ulster plan was to bring Protestant reform to the Irish Catholics. But the McIntosh family had not come to proselytize. Their motivation for leaving family, friends, and the only home they had ever known was far more pragmatic. It was the promise of replacing the heartbreak of rocky, unforgiving Scottish land with the rich, fertile Irish soil—it was the promise of a better life for their family.

They had settled near the village of Carrickfergus, on the north shore of Belfast Lough in County Antrim. Their closest neighbors were a family by the name of Hutchinson, who had come over from Ayrshire, Scotland, a few years earlier and established a successful farm. The Hutchinson clan had a large family with several strong sons who had helped the McIntosh clan clear their land for farming, raise a barn, and build a small stone house. The two families also helped establish a Presbyterian church in the community, which first met in their homes and later in a modest structure near the village green. They were a peace-loving congregation that coexisted comfortably with the other Christian denominations in the area. But, with all the hostility that swirled around them, it was hard to be sanguine in those early years.

The Irish Catholics had rebelled against the Protestant settlers for their anti-Catholic discrimination, leading to the Irish Rebellion of 1641 and the killing of thousands of English planters. In England it was referred to as the "Great Massacre." The fiercely anti-Catholic Cromwell led an English army to Ireland to seek revenge and take Ireland for England. It was one of the bloodiest times in Irish history. The McIntosh and Hutchinson families, along with most of the Scottish Presbyterians, were largely spared, although they grieved for the loss of their Catholic neighbors and lived in constant fear of what could happen to them.

During those fateful years, the McIntosh family established a general store in Carrickfergus to help supplement their farm income, and the current proprietor now stood behind his counter, watching the stranger as he moved among the wares. He judged the newcomer to be of middle age, with a slight stoop to his shoulders and a touch of gray in his light brown hair. He watched the man pick up a few items and then appear to be heading for the front door. Arthur moved quickly to head him off, but the stranger stopped at a table near the door and then casually turned to face his assailant with a disarming smile. The store keeper was flummoxed for a moment, and an awkward silence ensued until he regained his composure and spoke.

"Will ye be needin' anything more?" he asked, in a slightly accusatory tone.

The stranger looked down at the few items in his hands and was quiet and pensive for a second, then looked up, smiled again and shook his head.

"This will do for now, thank ye," he replied.

The two men walked over to the counter, where Arthur tallied up the cost of the items and announced it to his customer. The man nodded and reached into his pocket. Again, there was a tense moment as Arthur wondered whether the stranger was reaching for his money or a weapon. But the hand came out with a small number of coins, which were placed on the counter. The stranger looked up, and for the first time Arthur closely observed the features of his face. Not only was his smile disarming, but there was a peaceful and reassuring gaze in his hazel eyes.

John Leslie walked slowly down the dirt road from the general store with his bag in hand. The undertone of tension in the store had not escaped his notice, and he wondered if life here was going to be any better than that which he had left behind in Scotland. It had been the same the day before when he first arrived in the village. An official at the dock had given him the name of a person in town who rented rooms. When he arrived at the address, he had been met with the same circumspection that had just greeted him in the general store. The landlord was a native Irishman, by the name of Shields, whose Irish lineage extended back into the misty recesses of the country's history. Unlike most of the Irish, he was a Protestant, but he harbored the same suspicion that all his countrymen held for those coming over from the British Isles. He listened carefully to the accent of the stranger and seemed to relax a bit when he realized that he was Scottish and not English. He led John to a small upstairs room that contained only a bed, one straight chair, and a few hooks on the wall. And that would be his home in Ireland for the foreseeable future.

One week after his arrival in town, John again walked into the McIntosh General Store, although this time with a different purpose in mind. The store was empty except for the proprietor, who was in his usual position behind the counter. John did not make direct eye contact at first, but a side glance told him that he was still being closely scrutinized. He tried to appear casual and pretended to be checking out some items on a table. Then he looked over at Arthur McIntosh, smiled and took a few steps in his direction.

"John Leslie," he said, extending his hand.

"McIntosh, Arthur McIntosh." The response came with no change in expression on the proprietor's face, although he slowly offered his hand and was impressed by the firmness in the handshake of the man before him.

There followed a long, awkward silence, as both men looked down and seemed to be waiting for the other to speak. Finally, it was Arthur who broke the stillness.

"Saw ye at church last Sunday," he muttered, still looking down.

This brought an enthusiastic and sincere smile to John's face. He looked up with eager eyes and responded, "Aye, 'twas a lovely service, sure it was."

Arthur nodded in agreement and looked up into John's eyes for the first time that day, although his expression remained serious and still a bit reticent.

"From Scotland are ye?" he inquired.

"Aye. County Fife," John responded, as his smile faded, and he tried to affect the same serious demeanor as the proprietor.

"Leslie clan are ye?" the inquisition continued, still with no enthusiasm.

John nodded and began to worry about the direction the conversation was taking.

"Heard stories of thy kin," Arthur muttered, again looking down.

John didn't quite know what to make of that remark, but again nodded with a serious countenance, as though to say that he agreed with whatever it was that the proprietor was implying. There followed another long episode of discomfited silence, and again it was Arthur who finally spoke.

"Be there something I can do for ye?" he inquired, with puzzlement in his tone.

John wasn't quite sure at this point if he should continue with his mission or not. But a faint impression of friendliness in the storekeeper's last words gave him the courage to carry on.

"I saw the sign on thy door," he said with a timid, almost apologetic inflection.

The sign had not been there when John first visited the store, but he observed a few days later that a notice had been posted for the position of assistant clerk. Desperately needing to find work, he decided to give it a try. Arthur again looked up into John's eyes, this time as though he was attempting to ascertain the character of the man before him.

"Hast thou any experience?" he inquired.

"Aye, that I have," John responded, as he felt a bit of confidence— or at least hope—beginning to return. A slight nod from the proprietor, as though granting permission to proceed, encouraged him to do just that.

"Me family farmed and owned a general store in Scotland. When Father was killed in the war, me mother had to take over, and I did me best to help her as a lad. Eventually, I took charge and ran the store for her until she died. I sold it shortly before leavin' for Ireland."

For some time during their conversation, Arthur had been warming up to this new arrival. Not only did he feel the kinship of a fellow Scotsman and a Presbyterian, but he believed that he detected an assurance of honesty and integrity when he looked into his eyes. And now he saw the added attribute of the young man's past experience. And the truth was that, having just gotten rid of a rather worthless employee, he was much in need of good help.

John mulled over his thoughts for several agonizing moments. He had no way of knowing what was going through the older man's mind. He was about to apologize for bothering him and take his leave, when he saw Arthur smile for the first time.

"Well, lad, I'll give ye a week's trial and, if ye work be acceptable, we can talk about a long-term arrangement."

John had never felt such relief. A broad smile burst over his face, and he instinctively reached over the counter with both hands and enthusiastically shook the hand of his new boss.

Just then, another gentleman walked into the store. When Arthur saw him, his smile grew larger, and he blurted out a boisterous welcome.

"Angus Hutchinson, ye old scallywag, come over here and meet me new clerk."

Angus Hutchinson owned the farm adjacent to the McIntosh farm, and the two men had known each other for as long as either could remember. As young boys, they would hunt together in the woods and fish in the streams that wound through their parents' land. When they were old enough, they were both put to work in the family's potato fields. The day eventually came when each man took full responsibility for his farm. They stood together when their parents were buried in the common family cemetery, and they watched their children and grandchildren grow and assume increasing responsibilities within their families. They were in their sixties, but differed significantly in physical appearance. Arthur was bald and a bit shorter than average, with a stout frame and a full, ruddy face that was freely given to mirth. Angus was the more serious of the two, albeit with a dry wit; he was tall and slender, with an unruly shock of white hair that partially obscured a furrowed brow.

"Angus, meet John Leslie, newly arrived from County Fife," said Arthur McIntosh.

As the two men shook hands and maintained eye contact, John smiled, and Angus responded with a pleasant expression and a twinkle in his eye.

"So ye're going to work for this old horse thief are ye?" he asked, with the faintest hint of a smile.

"That be me hope, sir, but first I must prove me self," John replied with an uneasy smile, hoping that he was not misreading the apparent joshing of these two men, about whom he knew virtually nothing.

"Well, ye'll find him to be quite the slave driver, and see that ye never give thy back to him," Angus continued his banter.

"Angus, ye old reprobate," Arthur finally broke in, "might I be correct in supposin' that ye have come in to fleece me of a dram of me finest whiskey?" The fact was that Angus always dropped by the store at this late hour of the afternoon to share a small glass of Scotch whiskey with his best friend.

Angus feigned shock at such a question, but then revealed his first true smile of the day. The two older men laughed, and John soon joined in. They asked if he might like to raise a glass with them, to which he readily agreed. Arthur locked the front door and the men went to the back room of the store where they took their rest on three barrels, and the proprietor poured a round for each. Sitting there together at the end of the day—two old friends and their new acquaintance—none of them could have guessed how the winds of fortune would blow their three clans in paths that would cross and in places that they did not even know existed.

A lone bell pealed out from within the low, flat-topped steeple of the Presbyterian Church, bringing the faithful in wagons and on horseback, but mostly by foot. For nearly all of them, this was the most anticipated time of the week. It was a time to rest and a time to gather with friends and neighbors and catch up on the latest news. But, most importantly, it was a time to remember their blessings and to express their thanks through songs, scripture, prayer, and sermons. For John Leslie, it was all of those things and one more—a time to be near Molly.

Molly Hutchinson was Angus's youngest daughter and the only one yet to marry. At twenty-four, she was beyond the usual matrimonial age, and her father had begun to worry about her future. She was not a beauty, but there was something fetching in her delicacy. She was petite, and her most appealing feature was her complexion. She had delicate skin that was almost like white porcelain and was accented by her pale blue eyes. It was her striking, unvarnished complexion that she considered to be her best physical attribute, and she sought to enhance it by pulling her light brown hair back in a bun.

John appreciated Molly's appearance, but that was not what had drawn him to her. At church, he sat alone in the sanctuary, several rows back from the Hutchinson family and on the opposite side of the center aisle. This allowed him to observe Molly during the service, and what impressed him the most from the first time he noticed her was her sense of piety. When she prayed, she squeezed her eyes and often mouthed the words with intense sincerity. And, when she sang the hymns, it was as though she were communing with God himself, and a tear often slipped down her delicate cheek. John had always felt that the most important quality of the woman he would marry must be a faith that exceeded his own. And in Molly Hutchinson John felt that he had found such a woman.

For nearly six months, John admired Molly from afar, as his passion for her grew ever stronger and as he struggled to save enough from his earnings at the store to start a family. One day he finally mustered the courage to speak with Molly's father and ask his permission to begin courting his daughter. Angus tried to hide it, but his immense relief must have been apparent as he assured John that nothing could make him happier than to have him as a son-in-law. And so began the courtship of two mutually shy people, who would blush even to be seen holding hands. But it was evident to all that their love for each other was true, and it came as no surprise when they bashfully announced their engagement. And then, just when they were about to confirm their wedding date, an unthinkable tragedy struck.

John was working in the store when the town doctor came in to tell him that several cases of smallpox had recently been reported in a nearby community and that the epidemic was spreading in their direction. Being a doctor in those days could be very depressing, especially when their community was hit with an epidemic, such as smallpox, since there was so little help available for their patients. The best they could hope for was to prevent the spread of the disease by quarantining the afflicted and advising the others to take refuge in the country. Those with the disease suffered for many days with a high fever, generalized pain and fatigue, and pus-containing blisters on their face, limbs, and body. They often became delirious, and many died, while those who recovered were left with the telltale deep, pitted scars for the remainder of their life.

John felt that he was immune, having had a mild case in Scotland, but he was not sure about Molly. That evening, he walked over to the Hutchinson farm to discuss the matter. Angus and his wife had been exposed years before, but Molly and several others in the family had not. It was agreed that they should go to a small cabin on a hillside near a far corner of their property.

The days that followed were lonely ones for John, but he took comfort in knowing that his fiancée was safe and that they would soon be together forever when this threat had passed. He was especially thankful that Molly was in a safe haven when the epidemic hit Carrickfergus with a vengeance. After that, he didn't have much time to think about his loneliness, since he spent every waking hour, when he was not at the store, helping the doctor provide what little relief and comfort he could for the sick and dying. In all his intervening moments of solitude, he thought of Molly, thanked God that she was safe from the ravages of this horrible disease, and prayed for her continued well-being. But John was soon to be reminded that prayers are not always answered exactly as we wish.

He had just opened the store for the day when the doctor came in, accompanied by Angus Hutchinson. Both men bore long, dour faces, which was not uncommon during this episode of community crisis. But there was something more about their demeanor that made John uneasy. And, when they suggested that he come with them to the back room, he knew to brace himself for the worst.

The three men sat in silence for several long, anguishing minutes, as John's sense of anxiety and foreboding grew like a dark cloud filling the room. Finally, the doctor looked over at Angus, who closed his eyes for a moment and cleared his throat.

"John, I hate to be the one to tell ye this, but we ha'e just received word that our dear Molly hath been stricken with the smallpox."

John's first impulse was denial. Surely there must be a mistake. She had left town before the first case was discovered and had stayed away in a safe place. How could this happen? His heart was racing, and his mind was a muddle of anger and confusion. He turned to the doctor for answers.

"I know what ye be thinking," the doctor said, trying to control his own emotions. "We did all we could to protect her, sure we did, but we fear she may ha'e tried to help some poor soul along her way to the cabin and became exposed. You know Molly."

The doctor explained that Molly had been taken to another location, away from the others. They did not seem to want to tell him exactly where she was, and he did not press for any more answers. Angus told him that Molly's mother was with her and that everything possible was being done for her. There was nothing else they could do—except pray.

John did indeed pray. He had never prayed more fervently in all his life. He prayed day and night and slept very little. When brief, fitful sleep did come, he dreamed only of Molly, although too many of the dreams were nightmares. He would wake suddenly in a cold, anxious sweat and lie awake for the next hour praying that the vision he had just seen of himself standing alone in a cemetery was not a premonition of things to come. He went to work each day at the store, although he was only going through the motions, with his mind far off in another place. Townsfolk whom he had come to know as friends often came in to express their concern and to assure John that they were all praying for Molly.

Eventually, the last new case of smallpox in the town came and went, the epidemic began to recede, and the faithful filled their churches with prayers of gratitude. They also gave thanks for Molly, when word came that her fever had broken and the doctor predicted that she was going to live. Of course, no one gave thanks more passionately than a young man sitting in the back of the Presbyterian church. John spent every moment he could on his knees in front of the cross, with tears pouring down his cheeks as he thanked God with all his heart for sparing his dear Molly. His only thought now was being with her again as soon as possible. But his faith was about to be challenged more than at any time in his life.

When he was told the good news about Molly's recovery, John had first gone to the church to offer his gratitude and then to the Hutchinson farm to celebrate. But he was puzzled by a sense of silence and restraint among his future in-laws. John wondered why Molly was not home by now, since most other survivors in town were up and about. But he was told that she was still quite weak and needed more time before she could travel. So John waited, as days passed and then weeks, and he became more anxious and perplexed. He repeatedly inquired about her to Molly's parents. At first, they comforted him with assurance that she just needed more time, but the day came when he realized that there was something more that they were not telling him. On every visit, he beseeched them to let him know where she was, so he could go to her. But they always seemed to demur and change the subject. John was now even more distraught than when Molly had been sick; at least then he knew what was happening, but now he was totally at a loss to understand anything.

Angus seemed incapable or unwilling to even discuss it further with him, although Molly's mother finally admitted that her daughter was struggling with an overwhelming emotional uncertainty about her future. She was unsure of her feelings and thought she might even convert to the Catholic church and become a nun. John couldn't believe what he was hearing. He knew how much Molly wanted a family and children, and he was so sure of her love for him. There had to be more to it, he convinced himself. He poured his heart out to her in a letter that he asked Molly's mother to deliver. She took it and assured him that her daughter had received it, but no reply ever came.

Molly's parents could see how John was on the verge of insanity from the anguish that these inexplicable mysteries were causing him. And, in truth, they were not faring much better. Finally, Molly's mother could take it no longer and pretended to let it slip out as to where her daughter might be found. There was a small cottage tucked back in the hills just outside a nearby town, where they had some kindly friends.

The weather seemed to mirror John's mood as he trudged along the narrow dirt road, following the directions he had been given. The clouds overhead were dark, gloomy, and foreboding. In the distance, he could hear ominous peals of thunder, and he felt the wind beginning to pick up and rustle through the trees. Then, just as he turned to climb a winding path toward where he was told the cottage would be found, the heavens opened up with a cold rain that came down in torrents. Within seconds, he was soaked to the bone, and yet he barely noticed, so focused was he on his one mission. As he rounded the last bend in the path, he saw the little cottage. He had hoped to find a light in the window or some encouraging sign, but it was dark and unwelcoming, with no sign of life in the drab dwelling.

But there was someone inside. In a far corner of the dark, single room, a small figure sat with her back to the door holding her Bible—reading, praying, and crying. She did not hear the door open until a loud crash of thunder caused her to turn and see a rain-drenched man standing in the doorway, silhouetted by a bright flash of lightening. She screamed in fear, not recognizing her intruder. But the man did not move from the doorway and, as her eyes adjusted from the intensity of the lightening, Molly realized it was John. She instinctively turned her back to him, buried her face in her hands and began to cry bitterly, beseeching him to leave her.

John remained in the doorway for several long minutes, totally perplexed and dismayed by Molly's response to his arrival. Then he slowly closed the door and walked toward her. He placed a hand on her shoulder, which she pulled away, still unable to control her crying.

"Molly, what have I done to cause thy love for me to turn into this hatred?" he asked in a raspy voice, through emotions of his own that he could barely control.

He waited patiently for an answer, willing to give her all the time she needed. Finally, her crying abated long enough for her to take a deep, trembling breath and speak in a faint, whispered voice.

"I could never hate thee. Thou wilt always be my only love. But I am no longer worthy to be thy wife." The words came slowly and painfully between sobs and labored breathing.

John had no idea what she meant by that last phrase. But, as she remained seated with her back to him, seemingly unwilling to look at him, it finally began to dawn on him. He put his hands gently on her shoulders and turned her toward him. For a fleeting moment, she looked up into his face—the face she loved more than life itself—and then she hid her face in her hands and began crying again. And, in that instant, it all became clear to John, and he could barely keep from laughing in joyous relief. He wondered how he could have been so blind to have not seen it before.

In the moment that he had looked into her face, he saw the telltale scars of smallpox, which would forever be with her. Her lovely, unblemished skin—the only thing about her that she thought was beautiful—had been snatched from her, and she could no longer expect John to want her for his wife. But her love for him was so great that she did not want him to suffer the pain of being the one to call off the wedding—or, worse still, to go ahead with the wedding and live with someone that he could not love. But Molly had greatly underestimated the depth and purity of John's love for her.

They sat in silence for many long minutes, as Molly continued to cry with her face in her hands. John closed his eyes and asked for divine guidance to know what he should say to her. But he needn't have worried about finding the right words, because they poured from his heart.

"Dearest Molly, dost thou not know, I have loved thee with an everlasting love." His words were so tender and sincere that Molly thought her heart would surely break. Moreover, he was quoting one of her favorite Bible verses from the book of Jeremiah, and she understood what he was telling her—that his love for her was unconditional. She continued to cry, but now let him hold her in his arms, as tears also flooded his own eyes.

The morning dawned gloriously with a burst of sunshine. All the clouds had blown away overnight, and the countryside was washed clean and bright by yesterday's rain. The sky was clear blue, and the cheerful sunlight sparkled from raindrops that still clung to the trees and grass. From the cottage, a young couple emerged. In one hand, the man carried a lady's satchel, which had been hastily packed. In the other, he held the hand of his beloved. As they walked down the winding path, a profusion of wild flowers adorned their way, the birds serenaded them, and a gentle breeze flowed down from the hilltop, rustling the leaves above their heads and blowing lovingly at their backs.

Thus began the Leslies of Ireland. After their wedding, the young couple moved in with Molly's parents until they were able to build a modest home of their own on a small plot of land that Angus had helped them obtain near his farm. They worked hard to create a safe and loving environment, and soon there were little Leslies running around the homestead. With the rapidly expanding size of their family, more rooms were added to their house and many more acres to their farmland. For them, life was good, and they never failed to acknowledge the source of their blessings. But growing strife in the land continued to weigh heavily on them and their neighbors.

In the decades that followed John's arrival in Ireland, more Leslie families emigrated from Scotland to the Ulster Plantation. The majority survived the ongoing political upheavals, which were hardest on the Catholic population. But, as Ireland entered the eighteenth century, another threat was stealthily attacking the land, which showed no favoritism for political or religious persuasions and would eventually cause more devastation than anything the government could inflict. For more than a century, the Irish peasants had depended on their potato crops, which were easy to grow and required little land. But an unseen enemy, the potato blight fungus, soon began causing crop failures, with famines that, over the next two centuries, would cause millions to die or flee the country.

The first of the famines came in 1728, when John was in his eighty-seventh year. He and Molly had been blessed with a large family of children and grandchildren, all of whom were healthy and reasonably prosperous. But the crop failure caused John to worry about the future of his family more than with any of the country's previous crises. And yet he took comfort in knowing he had done all he could to prepare them for wherever the winds of fortune would blow.

For John, the winds were now blowing toward the place in which he had long since put his faith. He knew the time had come that he must leave his loved ones and all his future generations in the beneficent hands of Providence. In the fall of the year, as the last leaves drifted down from the old trees and blanketed the family farm, with Molly and all the family at his side and with a contented smile on his face, John Leslie breathed his last, his Bible in his hand.

CHAPTER 3

The Carolinas
1756–1807

THE LINE STRETCHED FOR AS FAR AS THE EYE COULD SEE. It inched along ridges that wound up steep slopes, passed through narrow gaps in mountains, and disappeared into hidden valleys. It reappeared beside serpentine riverbeds where flowing streams had carved out paths of least resistance over the ages. It went around or through dense woodlands and continued out into broad meadows until finally vanishing in thick clouds of dust.

The dust rose from a parched, rock-strewn trail, formed by countless pioneers who had passed that way in search of a better life and by the indigenous people who established the passageways long before the European settlers arrived. The dust was stirred up by the grinding of steel-rimmed wheels that supported all manner of wagons, buggies, and carts. It was kicked up by the hoofs of horses, oxen, and every type of livestock. And it rose from the feet of weary travelers, who trudged along in worn-out boots that provided little protection from the hot, sunbaked road or who continued their sojourn on bare, calloused feet.

Samuel Leslie was among the thousands in the long line of travelers who were heading south along the trace that skirted the Blue Ridge Mountains of the Virginia colony. Although his legs were aching and his feet were sore, he could not suppress a feeling of good fortune and optimism as he gazed at the beauty of the land that lay before him and the majesty of the distant, blue-tinged mountains that were his constant companions. But he worried about Sarah, who sat on the wooden seat of the wagon beside their five-year-old daughter. She had endured so many hardships since their marriage began, never complaining, and yet he wondered how much more she could take. He looked up at her, hoping for an encouraging smile, but saw only mind-numbing fatigue and a growing sense of despair on her weathered, dusty face.

It had been different when they first left Pennsylvania. Then there had been an air of excitement and confidence, and some were even laughing and singing as they set out on their latest quest for a better life. But that had been many weeks ago, and still there were many more to go before they reached their destination. Everyone was tired to the bone. Moreover, the supplies of food were running low, and there had been reports of illnesses among many of the families. There had even been a few burials along the way. And now they trudged on in silence, but with resolute determination written on their faces, and quite likely with many prayers in their hearts.

In their wagon, the Leslies carried all their worldly possessions. Among them, packed safely between a few items of clothing, was the family Bible. It was said that Samuel's great-grandfather had brought it over from Scotland nearly a hundred years ago. The leather binding was now cracked, and the corners were frayed. Most of the gold edging had long since worn off, and the metal latch no longer worked. But a signature of John Leslie was still legible on the front page, along with a date that indicated he was only a boy when he had signed it. Many other family names had since been added to the Bible, including those of Samuel's father and grandfather. It was a valuable record of his heritage, but much more, it was a symbol of the family's faith over the years and of their trust in the hand of Providence. Samuel had inherited his strong ancestral faith, yet he couldn't help but wonder if he had made the right decisions over those past hard years. Nothing had gone quite according to plan so far, and he worried about what lay ahead for his little family. Walking beside their wagon, day after day, his thoughts kept going back over the harrowing events that had brought them to this perilous juncture in their life.

Samuel had been born in County Antrim between the first and second crop failures to hit the Ulster region of Ireland in the eighteenth century. He was only five when the second famine came, in 1740, but he could recall how it devastated their community. He was vaguely aware that some people had died because they did not have enough to eat and that others had just disappeared. What he remembered most vividly was people coming to his parents' farm, some of whom he had never seen before, begging for food. His father had planted other crops in addition to their potatoes, and they were a little better off than many of their neighbors. They did what they could to help the less fortunate, although Samuel realized that it left his family with barely enough to survive during that trying year. It seemed that they had just recovered from the latest famine when another potato blight led to a crop failure four years later. For some, this was the final blow, and an ever-increasing number of families began leaving Ireland, many going to a place that his parents called the New World.

One of the Leslies' nearest neighbors and closest friends were the Hutchinsons. They were one of several Hutchinson families in the area, and were distantly related to the Angus Hutchinson family, whose daughter, Molly, was Samuel's great-grandmother. The Hutchinsons were linen weavers and lived near the village of Carrickfergus on the shore of Belfast Lough. They had six daughters, the fifth of whom they named Sarah. Samuel and Sarah had known each other since they were old enough to remember, but it was not until they were in their teens that they began to see each other as more than just playmates. Samuel began courting Sarah, and they were married as he approached his twentieth year. That proved to be bad timing, as a fourth crop failure and famine hit Ireland the following year, in 1756. It would be the first of many challenges for the young couple, who had to turn to their parents for help, but even they were barely able to make ends meet. The repeated crop failures, combined with periodic depression in the linen trade and attacks on Presbyterianism, had caused up to 10,000 Scotch-Irish to leave the Ulster region each year during the middle of the century. Samuel and

Sarah had already begun talking with some of their siblings about joining the vast migration to America, and the latest crop failure convinced them that the time had come.

But the decision to leave home and family for such a distant, unknown land, with little prospect of ever returning, was the hardest thing that either of them ever had to do. And they might have backed out altogether were it not for the fact that three of Sarah's sisters, Grace, Jane, and Mary, would be going with them. In addition, Samuel's brother, John, who was courting Mary, had decided to join the little band of travelers. Even so, there were many hours of discussion and prayer among the two families before it was finally settled. Their parents knew there was no future for the young people in Ulster and, as heartbreaking as it was for them, they had to agree that their children were better off seeking their fortune in the New World.

And so, on a cold, drizzling morning before daybreak, the Leslie and Hutchinson families crowded into two wagons and left Carrickfergus for the short drive beside the lough down to the harbor of Belfast, where a schooner sat rigged and waiting. For Samuel and Sarah, that moment on the dock, saying goodbye to their parents, knowing they might never see them again, would forever be among their most anguished memories. And yet at the same time they would recall a sense of exhilaration as they walked up the gangplank of the shiny vessel, with its huge sails flapping overhead in the gentle breeze, wondering where the winds of Providence might take them. The six young people stood at the railing, waving to their families, as the ship slowly edged away from the dock and headed up the lough toward the Irish Sea. They continued waving until the last person on the dock was shrouded in the late morning fog, and then they stood in silence, each wondering if they had made the right decision.

Ocean travel in those days was an uncomfortable and unpleasant experience at best. The quarters were cramped, poorly ventilated, and musty. Passengers generally had to provide their own food and just hoped it would last the voyage. And there was always the agony of seasickness. At its worst, sailing on the open seas was downright dangerous. The masted ships were at the mercy of the elements—the wind, the sea states, and the sudden storms that could throw a ship off course or even sink it. Added to that was the ever-present danger of pirates on the high seas. The young Leslies and Hutchinsons were, fortunately, naïve about most of these disadvantages of ocean travel as they headed out on their journey, but they would learn soon enough.

As the ship sailed up Belfast Lough, the water was calm, and the young people began to think that sailing was going to be rather pleasant after all. But when the ship turned south into the Irish Sea between Ireland and the British Isles, the waves began to rise, and the vessel began the rhythmic undulations the would be the traveler's bane for the remainder of the journey. At first, there seemed to be an element of adventure in the ship's movement, and the six young sojourners chatted merrily. Before long, however, a silence overtook their party, and they began to look at one another, wondering if the others were experiencing the same unpleasant feeling of nausea. And the worst was yet to come.

Their ship continued south for the rest of the first day. It was nighttime before it rounded the southern tip of Ireland and headed west into the Atlantic Ocean. None of the young people had eaten much that first day, and they were all thankful to lie down in their bunks when evening came to achieve some relief from their seasickness. The motion of the ship actually seemed rather calming at first and lulled most of them into a restless sleep. Sometime during the night, however, they were all awakened by violent movement of the ship and terrifying crashing sounds. Samuel struggled to the deck to inquire of a crew member, feeling certain that they must have encountered a major storm. But the crewman just laughed and said, "Welcome to the Atlantic, mate."

Over the days that followed, things did not get much better. Samuel and John partially overcame their motion sickness and were able to spend some time together on deck, but the four women stayed in their beds for nearly the entire trip, eating very little. Sarah seemed to suffer the most, being able to hold down only small sips of water, and Samuel became gravely concerned and prayed constantly for her health. At one point, in the middle of the Atlantic, they hit a true storm, sending everyone to bed and holding tight to whatever they could to keep from rolling onto the floor. But, as bad as it seemed for the six young travelers, the crew called it an uneventful voyage, and on a clear, sunny day they finally sailed into the relatively calm water of Delaware Bay. From there, the ship turned north to a landing near the settlement of New Castle on the Delaware River.

Sarah was so weak that Samuel had to carry her off the ship. He found lodging near the wharf, where he nursed her back to a semblance of health, all the while nursing his own guilt for having put his young wife through such an awful experience. He prayed that things would soon get better, but it was just as well that he didn't know what lay around the next bend.

Pennsylvania colony was a popular destination for many of the Scotch-Irish who emigrated from Ulster. Founded by the Quaker William Penn, it offered a haven for religious dissenters who practiced what many considered to be unorthodoxy. However, being of modest means, most of the Scotch-Irish headed for the backcountry, in and around the town of Lancaster, about fifty miles northwest of New Castle as the crow flies. Samuel and John were able to buy a used wagon, and, when Sarah was well enough to travel, they packed all their worldly belongings in the back of the wagon, and the six of them headed out for their new life in the backcountry of Lancaster, Pennsylvania.

When they arrived, they quickly learned the meaning of the word "backcountry." It was the closest thing to the fringes of civilization that any of them had yet experienced. But at least they were with people of their own ethnic and religious background, and there was a small Presbyterian church, which for Samuel was the most important prerequisite in finding their new home. On their first night near Lancaster, the six young people went into the chapel of the church and knelt together before the cross, held hands, and fervently thanked God for bringing them safely thus far on their long, perilous journey.

Good-hearted people from the church shared their modest dwellings with the newcomers until Samuel and John were able to build a primitive one-room house into which all six of them crowded. They planted crops on a small plot of land that they were able to acquire and soon added a second room to their home so that Samuel and Sarah could have a bit of privacy. Before long, it was necessary to add yet a third room, as John and Mary announced their plans for a wedding. That was the first of several joyous occasions for the Leslies and Hutchinsons in the strange new land that they now called home. The second came the following year, when Sarah gave birth to their first child. They named her Sarah, after her mother, although some called her Sally to keep the two straight. In the meantime, Jane had met a young man named James Crawford, whose father had come over from Ayrshire, Scotland, and soon the families were celebrating yet another wedding. Those events would be remembered as the highlights of their years in Pennsylvania. But another event was casting a dark shadow over all the community around Lancaster, which would eventually bring this phase of their life to an end.

Many Native American tribes had lived for ages in and around the land that Europeans now called Pennsylvania. Most were peaceful and were willing to coexist with the first settlers to arrive, even helping some get started in their new home. But, as more settlers came into the area and showed little inclination to share the land, the tribes began to realize that their ancient way of life was in jeopardy. When they learned that the Europeans were also divided into tribes, with England and France being the main ones, they devised a strategy of playing one against the other. Several tribes, most notably the Delaware and Shawnee, allied with the French and launched campaigns of terror on British settlements in the Ohio Valley. England retaliated by forming their own alliances with local tribes, including the Iroquois, which led to a drawn-out conflict that the British called the French and Indian War.

The War began in 1754, two years before the Leslies and Hutchinsons arrived in America, and continued for nine years, culminating in the French surrendering all their North American territories. With the official cessation of formal hostilities, the settlers hoped to enjoy a time of peace, but the dangers they faced only seemed to escalate. England had shown little or no interest in rewarding the tribes that had aided them in their victory, and now all the Indians in the area had to confront the reality that they were losing the land. Some gave up and moved further west, but many stayed and defended their land in the only way they knew how—with periodic raids that they hoped would discourage further settlements. And the settlers to be hit hardest were those living in the backcountry.

Samuel and John peered nervously through cracks in the window of their home. In sweaty, shaking hands they held their rifles, which they had never used for anything except hunting game to feed their families. Sarah hugged her young daughter and tried to comfort her, as she and her sisters cowered in the far, dark corner of the room, trembling and crying. Samuel could not believe that he had once again put his wife, and now their daughter, in such peril.

Through the crack, Samuel could see fire coming from a house that was less than a quarter mile away. He could make out figures on horseback and hear shouting and gunshots. His heart was racing, and his eyes stung from the perspiration pouring from his brow, as he steeled himself to protect his family if the conflagration came any closer. But just as quickly as it had come, it suddenly seemed to be over. There was a long, eerie silence, and then he heard a neighbor's voice calling for every able-bodied man to come help. Samuel and John first made sure the women were safe, and then went to help put out the fire and attend to the wounded. When they returned to their house, all of them sat together for the remainder of the night, talking and praying.

Many of their neighbors had already left, joining the ever-growing number of wagon trains that were heading south, in the hope of finding not only a greater abundance of fertile land but also a safer place for their families to live. As they had done less than a decade before in Ireland, the Leslies and Hutchinsons had once again begun trying to divine the best course for their future. But the harrowing events of that black night left them with no doubts.

As the wagon train continued through Virginia, Samuel became increasingly agitated, thinking back over all the agony and danger that he had caused his young family: the heartbreak of leaving their parents in Ireland, the perils and distress of travel on the open sea, the backbreaking work of building a new home under the constant threat of war and violence, and now this seemingly endless trek to yet another unknown place that he had no assurance would be any better. As he was painfully reliving those agonizing years, he felt something gently rest on his shoulder, and he looked up to see Sarah gazing down at him with a tired but comforting smile. She seemed to know when he was in one of his self-flagellating moods, and she had a way of easing his mind like a soothing balm. As Samuel looked at his wife, he realized how blessed he was to have her by his side, and for the moment all his cares seemed to evaporate, like feathers blowing away in a gentle breeze.

Looking up into his wife's exhausted but determined face, he could still see traces of the delicate young woman he had married a decade ago. Her tender lips were now cracked and dried, but still capable of the loving smile that had won his heart. Her once smooth skin was brown and leathery from years of exposure to the elements, but her high cheekbones and the graceful curve of her nose still gave her a timeless beauty. Her auburn hair, tucked beneath a straw bonnet, rarely received much attention these days, but loose ends danced in the wind and reflected red highlights in the afternoon sunlight. And the one part of her beauty that would never fade was her soft brown eyes that looked down at her husband and bespoke gentleness, strength, faith, and love.

Just then, they heard a commotion far up the line ahead of them. A bugle was blowing, and men were shouting. His first thought was that it might be an Indian raid. He had been told that such attacks occurred on the trail, although they had been mercifully spared thus far. But, as the shouting voices drew closer to their position, he began to understand the message that was being relayed from one wagon to the next—they had just crossed the border into North Carolina.

By the time their wagons reached the line, the sun was hanging low in the sky with a warm, golden glow. It cast long shadows across the trail in front of them and painted the groves of pine trees with streaks of brilliant orange light. Samuel had assumed that there would be no noticeable difference in the landscape when they crossed from Virginia into North Carolina, and yet there did seem to be a difference. The mountain range that had accompanied them for most of their trek through Virginia was now far behind them, and the open grasslands were giving way to densely wooded, rolling hills. The pine trees stood tall and stately, with their straight, bare trunks leading up to thick boughs of green needles. Deep in the woods, hemlocks and hickory trees, dogwoods and redbuds, mingled with the tall pines, and a thick bed of pine needles gave the air a fragrant, pungent aroma. A gentle breeze rustled through the pine boughs high overhead, causing the shafts of orange sunlight to sparkle down through the trees and across the dense ground cover and the road that lay ahead of the weary but heartened travelers.

Having reached North Carolina, it felt as though their long journey was near an end. And yet, more than 200 miles still lay ahead of them. Their destination was along the South Carolina border, where some of their extended family had already settled. Jane and her husband, James, had left Lancaster shortly after their marriage, and the Crawfords had established a homestead near the border between the two Carolinas. Sarah's oldest sister, Margaret, had married a Scotch-Irish man by the name of George McKemey while they were still living in Ireland. George had come to America alone and started a prosperous farm near the Crawfords before bringing Margaret. Sarah and her two sisters were giddy with excitement over the prospect of soon being reunited with Jane and Margaret.

The first town of any size that Samuel and his family reached in North Carolina was Hillsborough, in the northern Piedmont section of the colony. They were relieved to find a semblance of civilization in the small community and spent several days there, resting, restocking their provisions, and gathering information about the next leg of their journey. Samuel and John enjoyed chatting with the local townsmen. Even though there were some grumblings about the arrogance of the royal governor, the two brothers sensed an air of excitement about the prospects for a good life in this new part of the world. And there were certainly many who seemed to share this feeling of optimism about the future of the Carolinas. One of the men in Hillsborough told Samuel that, in the past year, he had counted over a thousand wagons passing through their town on the way to points south.

After Hillsborough, the trail turned west toward the settlement of Salisbury. They were now traveling through the heart of North Carolina, crossing rivers, passing through valleys and over hills that were becoming ever larger as they drew nearer to the great Western mountains. They traversed dense woodlands, where giant trees blocked out much of the sunlight, and then came into open meadows, where lonely farms could be seen off in the distance. Most of the civilization they saw was the isolated farms and occasional clusters of homes that would one day become villages. Samuel had been told that this was the frontier, and he felt that he was beginning to understand the difference between backcountry and frontier. In the backcountry of Pennsylvania, there had seemed to be a survival mentality and a sense of defiance against authority. The people wanted to be left alone and to scratch out a living in whatever way they could manage. But, on the frontier of the Carolinas, Samuel sensed a feeling of optimism—of people pulling together to create something new and better for themselves and for those who would come after them. That thought filled him with exhilaration and hope for the future of his family. And his optimism was only enhanced when Sarah presented him with the latest family news.

She had not been feeling well in Hillsborough, with headaches and episodes of nausea and vomiting, especially in the morning hours. She was fairly sure of the cause but decided not to say anything until she was certain. Seeing how concerned Samuel was about her health, she decided that the time had come. And so, on a warm evening, when they had stopped to camp for the night between Hillsborough and Salisbury, Sarah informed her husband that they would be having their second child shortly after settling in their new home. Samuel couldn't wait to tell the others, and there was general celebration that evening. Of course, they were all concerned about her traveling in that condition, but they knew that, if anyone could manage, it was Sarah.

Before they had left Ireland, Sarah had developed a keen interest in the healing arts. It was not so much the scientific aspects that appealed to her, as the humanitarian. Whenever someone in Carrickfergus was ill, she would invariably do whatever she could to bring comfort and relief, not only to the patient but to all the family. Her greatest satisfaction came from attending young women in labor. She observed closely how the older women assisted in the delivery and paid special attention when the doctor came to manage complicated cases. Before long, this apprenticeship led to her being recognized throughout the community as a skillful and trusted midwife.

They spent a week in the Salisbury camp, until the expectant mother felt well enough to start on the final leg of their journey. The trail now divided in two directions: one continuing west toward the mountains, and the other turning south toward the South Carolina border. The Leslie and Hutchinson party took the latter route to where family waited for them in a settlement called Waxhaw. It had been founded about a decade earlier along Waxhaw Creek just east of the Catawba River. Both the valley and the river that ran through it had been named after the Catawba Indians, a relatively young tribe that had been formed as an amalgamation of ancestral tribes of the Piedmont that had been decimated by disease and wars. But Samuel and Sarah's relatives had sent encouraging words about the beauty and fertility of the land and the peacefulness of its inhabitants. And that buoyed the spirits of the little band of weary travelers as they anticipated finally reaching their destination.

As they headed south, paralleling the course of the Catawba River, Samuel noticed a subtle change in the air. There was a hint of coolness in the wind that rustled the leaves overhead. It seemed to be heralding a transition of seasons. And there were new wildflowers along the roadside, with blossoms of golden yellow, lacy white, and deep purple. And those leaves rustling in the trees were losing their dark green hues for warm tints of yellow, orange, and russet. As their wagons drew near to Waxhaw, they passed fields where hay was stacked like pyramids and bright orange pumpkins were collected on the tilled soil. By now, there was a decided chill to the air, and the trees were reaching their full autumn glory. It seemed as though the land was welcoming them to their new home, and the young travelers felt a profound sense of good fortune, as each silently offered up prayers of thanksgiving.

Margaret was working in their garden when she saw the wagons approaching their farm. She shouted to George, who was in the field behind his mule, and then dropped her trowel and began running toward the road. Grace was the first to jump from the wagon and begin racing toward her sister, with Mary close behind. Sarah wanted desperately to join them but knew she would have to be patient for a few more minutes. When the four sisters were finally all together, the tears flowed freely as they hugged and kissed and laughed and wept. Shortly, George McKemey arrived from the field and solemnly shook hands with the two Leslie brothers. The three men tried to maintain their manly composure, but they too had difficulty holding back a tear.

That evening, they all paid a surprise visit to Jane and James Crawford, whose farm was about three miles south of the McKemeys. There were more tears and hugging and laughter, as Jane was reunited with her three sisters for the first time in so many years. They all sat around a crackling fire that evening. Little Sally, who had been such a trouper throughout the long trek, soon drifted off to sleep against her mother's shoulder, but the adults stayed up, talking into the wee hours of the morning. There was so much to tell and so many things to discuss and so many plans to make. With winter coming on, it was agreed that Samuel Leslie's family would stay with the McKemeys, and John, Mary, and Grace would spend the winter with the Crawfords.

The Leslie brothers helped George and James bring in their harvests that fall and prepare their farms for the winter. They also surveyed land in the surrounding area, looking for sites where they could start their own farms in the spring. Before long, the first snows of winter began to blanket the land with pristine white glory. Inside the two farmhouses, there was warmth and coziness and the love of family reunited. On Christmas Eve, they all attended the candlelight service at the Waxhaw Presbyterian meetinghouse. In the warm glow of the candles, they bowed their heads and offered sincere thanks for God's grace in bringing them safely through their perilous journey to a land that offered such promise for the future of their families.

They were pleasantly surprised to find how early spring came to the Carolinas. By late February, tender shoots were already breaking through winter's last crusty remnant of snow, and blue and yellow blossoms soon brightened an otherwise dreary countryside. Within weeks, small trees were bursting forth with white, pink, and purple blossoms that were soon followed by the light green blush of new leaves. The cold chill of winter was giving way to warm, sunny days, and gentle breezes carried the fragrance of the flowers and the lilting melodies of the songbirds. Like every young man throughout time, Samuel was invigorated by the arrival of spring. He couldn't wait to get outside, dig in the ground, plant his first crops, and begin to build a home for his little family.

Over the winter, Samuel had found a suitable site for their farm, which was about a half mile southeast of the McKemey homestead. It was agreed that the four men would first focus on putting up a modest house and some outbuildings on this new land, in consideration of Sarah's impending motherhood. The timing was good, as the house was barely completed when Sarah gave birth to their first son. They named him John, after his uncle and his great-great-grandfather, who had brought their lineage over from Scotland. He was a strong, healthy baby and brought immense joy to his parents and his sister and all their extended family in the Waxhaw Valley. But for the five Hutchinson sisters there was still one thing lacking to make their joy complete—to be reunited with Elizabeth.

Elizabeth Hutchinson was the youngest of the six sisters and the last to leave Ireland. She was short and plump, with blue eyes, red hair, and an indomitable spirit, which she would need in spades for the challenges that life was to throw at her. In Carrickfergus, there was a family by the name of Jackson, who lived near the Leslies and Hutchinsons. Elizabeth fell in love with their son Andrew, and the young couple married and soon had two sons, Hugh and Robert. When the boys were one and three years of age, the family set out in the footsteps of Elizabeth's sisters—a perilous trans-Atlantic crossing and disembarking along the Delaware River. But they immediately headed south with the wagon trains through Virginia and into the

Carolinas. It all seemed worth the cost when Elizabeth was joyfully reunited with her sisters—the first time all six had been together in over a decade.

Andrew Jackson found a wooded acreage about six miles north of the Samuel Leslie farm along Twelve Mile Creek, where he built their home and worked tirelessly to clear the land and plant his crops. They had been in the Carolinas for a little over a year when Elizabeth informed Andrew that, come springtime, they would be welcoming their third child. He greeted the news with typical fatherly pride and joy, but also with a redoubled dedication to provide for their growing family. He first had to tend and harvest the crops, and then he turned to clearing more land to expand next year's plantings. By now, winter was setting in, with cold rains and occasional snows, but Andrew continued his relentless, exhausting labor. One night he came into the house, barely able to stand or talk. He was having difficulty breathing and told Elizabeth that he had a crushing pain in his left shoulder. They both hoped a good night of sleep would be the answer. But, in the morning, Andrew was unable to get out of bed.

Elizabeth knew now that something was seriously wrong with her husband. She hurriedly hitched their horse to the wagon and, leaving Hugh to watch over his father, she and Robert drove as fast as they could to Samuel Leslie's farm. Sarah went back to the Jackson farm with Elizabeth and Robert, while Samuel saddled his horse and rode to the nearest town that had a doctor. When the two women entered the house, they found Andrew still in bed, covered in perspiration, with labored breathing and barely able to speak. Sarah put her hand on his forehead, which seemed to be on fire. She asked Elizabeth to bring cold, wet cloths and put them on his head and chest to reduce the fever. Then they sat beside him, waiting for the doctor to arrive and praying.

The doctor was typical of the available medical care on the frontier—limited education and even more limited resources. But what he lacked in knowledge and skill, he made up for in dedication and compassion. It was early afternoon before he walked into the Jacksons' one-room home. As he sat beside Andrew, feeling his pulse and his forehead, Sarah could see on his face the look of frustration and despair that she had seen so many times before on the faces of the healers. She often wondered what it was that enabled them to carry on against such formidable and discouraging odds, but she was just thankful that there were those who were willing to do what they could to relieve suffering.

The doctor told the women that Andrew had an infection in his lungs and that his heart was strained and laboring. He could only provide some medication for comfort, but he had nothing to treat his breathing or his struggling heart. He stayed beside his patient through the afternoon and into the evening, while the family waited in the background, crying and praying. At one point it seemed that Andrew might be improving, as his breathing relaxed, but the doctor knew better. He held Andrew's wrist for a long time, then leaned his ear near his patient's mouth and nose. Finally, he gently laid Andrew's arm across his chest and slowly pulled the sheet over his face. With two young boys to care for and a third child on the way, Elizabeth suddenly realized that she was a widow.

She stayed in their home on Twelve Mile Creek that winter, hoping she and her boys might be able to keep the farm going. January ushered in the year 1767, and by mid-March Elizabeth knew her third child was about to enter the world. Again she rigged the family wagon and, with the boys in the back, headed out for the Crawfords' home, where it had been agreed that she would give birth to her baby, with Sarah serving as the midwife. However, as the contractions grew stronger, she realized that she wasn't going to make it that far and detoured to the McKemey farm. Sarah was notified and arrived just in time to assist Elizabeth in giving birth to her third son. In honor of his recently departed father, the child was given the name Andrew.

With an infant and two rambunctious young boys to care for, Elizabeth soon realized that it was not going to be possible for her to maintain the farm. Of her five sisters, Jane and her husband, James, were the most prosperous. In addition, Jane had become a semi-invalid who was having difficulty running their home and caring for their several children. And so it was that Elizabeth and her three boys moved in with the Crawfords, where she took over the running of the household.

For Samuel and Sarah Leslie, the years flew by. They had two more sons, Robert and George, and another daughter, Mary. Their oldest son, John, was close in age to his three Jackson cousins, and the boys had enjoyed playing together since they were old enough to remember. However, since their farms were several miles apart, they usually saw each other only on Sundays. And, for active, young boys, those days had their pluses and minuses. They loved the time they had to run and play ball and explore areas around the meetinghouse. But sitting on hard pews during long services was another matter. The Presbyterian order of worship in those days was rather austere and rigid. Services typically started around midmorning with the singing of a psalm—without instrumental accompaniment—followed by a lengthy prayer. Then came a scripture lesson, the minister's sermon, and another psalm. The whole thing lasted about two hours, which seemed like an eternity for the young boys. But what kept their spirits up was the anticipation of the lunch that would follow and then some time to run and play. In the afternoon, there was another two-hour service, and then a little more time for the children to play, while the adults stood around and chatted. Finally, as long shadows began to stretch across the churchyard, the families would load into their wagons, wave goodbye, and head home.

When John Leslie was young, he especially enjoyed the companionship of his cousin Andy, who was exceptionally bright and full of energy and fun. Elizabeth had hopes that her youngest son would one day enter the ministry, and she arranged lessons for him with a Presbyterian clergyman. But, as Andy grew older, it became increasingly apparent to his mother and everyone else that he was not destined to be a man of the cloth. He had a feisty stubborn streak, an almost unmanageable will, and a defiant temper. This attitude was anathema to John's personality, and he made an effort to avoid his cousin more and more as they grew older. Samuel Leslie predicted that Andrew would quite likely never make it through childhood, but that if he did survive to manhood, there was no limit as to what he might accomplish.

As another January ushered in a new decade, conversations around Waxhaw were turning increasingly to the British government and the injustices it was imposing on the colonies. In the spring of 1771, word came of a tragedy near the settlement of Alamance, not far from Hillsborough, where Samuel and his party had stopped on their trek south. A group of North Carolinians in the Piedmont had formed a group called the Regulators in opposition to what they saw as unjust and corrupt laws of Governor Tryon. On a Saturday in late May, they had met beside Alamance Creek for a peaceful protest, when Tryon and his militia showed up and ordered them to disperse. Shots were fired and lives were lost on both sides, before the Regulators retreated into the woods. Tryon arrested some of their leaders, several of whom were tried and hanged.

Few in Waxhaw doubted that this incident was a harbinger of worse things to come, and they were not surprised when, four years later, word came of further skirmishes with the British, this time to the north in towns called Lexington and Concord. As conflict, which American history would record as the Revolutionary War, now seemed inevitable, the people of Waxhaw, like those throughout the colonies, became divided in their allegiance. Samuel had every reason to hate the British for the way they had treated the Scots and the Irish, but his overriding concern was to avoid more bloodshed. For that reason, he somewhat reluctantly leaned toward the Loyalist side of George III, feeling that Britain had the best chance of bringing a quick conclusion to the conflict. But many in his community sided with the Whigs, who cast their lot with the Continental Congress, and some of those were his own relatives living in the Crawford household. Andy Jackson's oldest brother, Hugh, joined the rebels for a brief moment of glory. He died—reportedly of heat and exhaustion—during a battle near Charleston. As the war relentlessly dragged on, it expanded into the south, especially the Carolinas and Georgia, where some of the most brutal fighting would occur. In 1780, British troops under the command of a Lt. Col. Tarleton staged an attack near Waxhaw, killing 130 men and wounding 150 more in a gruesome carnage that earned their leader the name "Bloody Tarleton."

Samuel realized now that he could no longer support the British, but he tried to maintain an appearance of neutrality in an attempt to protect his family, which was mercifully spared. Others in the community, however, were less fortunate, and among those were his relatives in the Crawford household. A small British force trapped Andy and Robert in their home, where they savagely beat the boys and marched them off to a British prison camp about forty miles away in Camden. When Elizabeth learned of her sons' situation, she walked the forty miles to the prison and pleaded with the British for the release of her boys. Her petition was finally granted, and the three Jacksons walked home, with the boys in bare feet, through freezing, wet weather. Both brothers had suffered severe head injuries when they were attacked in their home. Andrew's eventually healed with a permanent scar, but Robert's developed an infection, which spread to his brain. As Elizabeth sat in the Crawfords' home trying to comfort her feverish, disoriented son, she could only watch and cry and pray as her second child slowly slipped away from her.

And yet her indomitable spirit would not allow her to give up. After nursing Andrew back to health, she volunteered at a hospital in Charleston, where she cared for the sick and dying soldiers. While there, she contracted a fatal illness from one of her patients. And so it was that a remarkable woman, who had left her home in Ireland, braved the perils of the high seas and wagon trains, and lost her husband and two of her three sons, died in obscurity in the fall of 1781 and was buried in an unmarked grave. Many years later, Andrew Jackson, seventh president of the United States, would return in search of his mother's grave site, but to no avail.

The people of Waxhaw were never quite the same after the Revolutionary War. Every single person had been touched by the killing, the destruction, the pain and sorrow, and the constant fear. There were no victory celebrations when word filtered south that the British were going home. Some of the families that had remained Loyalist left the settlement, possibly returning to the old country; others just remained quiet. For the rest, there was a reserved sense of optimism and of hope that their new government would bring a better way of life. And all the faithful gathered in their churches to pray for the souls of those who had perished, to thank God for those who had been spared, and to entreat the Almighty for guidance as their fledgling nation ventured into the great unknown.

The years continued to march on, and the scars of war gradually began to heal. John Leslie grew to manhood, but remained on his parents' farm, taking an increasingly heavy load of the work and responsibilities. In the final decade of the eighteenth century, he met a young lady named Jane McElwee, whose family history was remarkably similar to his own—emigration from Scotland to Ireland to the New World, and a brief time in Pennsylvania before moving to South Carolina, where her family established a prosperous farm not far from the Samuel Leslie homestead. They were also devout Presbyterians.

John and Jane fell in love and were married in the spring of 1792. The young couple settled on the McElwee farm, and there the family grew rapidly, with eight children by 1806. The country was also expanding, and the direction of the expansion was shifting from southward to westward, as land became increasingly scarce in the southern states. The United States, under President Jefferson, had purchased a vast tract of land from France, which extended the boundaries of the country further south and far to the west. Young people were being advised to take advantage of the fertile and plentiful land that lay out west. And one of the recommended destinations was the nascent state of Kentucky.

While John and Jane were happy living on the McElwee farm and grateful to share the good life that their family enjoyed, they longed to have a place of their own. One evening, John came home with a paper in his hand and an excited expression on his face, and Jane had a feeling that their life was about to change. The paper told of affordable land in a part of Kentucky called Barren County. They stayed up late that night, reading and rereading the encouraging reports about the life that awaited those with the courage to move west. And the next day John drove over to his father's farm for a serious talk.

As Samuel Leslie sat on the porch of his farmhouse, looking out across the Carolina landscape and listening to his son talk about the future, his mind drifted back some fifty years to a time when he was a young man in Carrickfergus, talking with his father and mother about his own future. And, at that moment, he understood how his

parents must have felt as they faced the loss of their loved ones—
the heartbreak of knowing that they might never see them again,
that they would not be able to watch their children succeed in life or
watch their grandchildren grow up, that they would not be there for
births and birthdays, for baptisms and weddings, and for funerals.
Of course, Kentucky was not nearly as far away as the New World
had been from Ireland, but it was far enough by the transportation
of the day that Samuel realized he would likely never see John and
his family again.

John could see that his father was struggling with his emotions,
and he wondered how much he had actually heard of his plans. He
allowed several minutes of silence to pass, as the two men stared off
toward the hills on the horizon, before he spoke again.

"Well, Pa, what do ya think?"

The silence that followed was even longer. Samuel had a distant,
melancholy look as he continued to gaze off at nothing in particular.
He had read the papers also and knew of the opportunities that
waited out west for those who were willing to accept the risks and
do the hard work. He also remembered the feelings he had had as a
young man—the sense of exhilaration and anticipation for what lay
out there in faraway places. Without averting his gaze, but with a
lump in his throat, he finally offered his opinion.

"Well, son, ya gotta follow where yer heart leads ya."

And so, on a clear spring day in 1807, two large wagons sat rigged
and packed at the McElwee farm. The sky was blue and cloudless,
the sunshine was warm, and the breeze was gentle and cool. All the
Leslie and McElwee families had gathered for the sendoff. In the
front wagon, John sat on the driver's bench with his daughters, Mary
and Elizabeth, beside him. In the wagon behind him, his oldest son,
George, who was now fourteen but big for his age, held the reins.
Beside him sat his mother, holding one-year-old Grace, while the
other four children, William, Margaret, John, and Jane, snuggled
together in the back among their family's possessions.

There had been prayers and tears and hugs and a reluctance to
let go, but the two wagons finally pulled out, amid much waving
and shouts of love and best wishes. Those remaining behind stood

for a long time, watching the wagons disappear toward the horizon. One by one, they returned to their homes, until finally Samuel and Sarah were left alone, watching a cloud of dust as it settled beyond a distant hill. Each knew what the other was thinking—of a young couple on a similar venture nearly fifty years earlier and all that had happened since that time, and of the empty feeling that their parents must have felt then and which tore at their hearts now.

They stood there together for a long time, holding hands, as the tears began to dry. Sarah gave Samuel's hand a gentle squeeze and glanced up at him with her loving smile, as she had once done so long ago. And Samuel felt a comforting breeze encircle them.

CHAPTER 4

Arkansas
1838–1886

D URING THE FIRST HALF of the nineteenth century, long lines of humanity could once again be seen winding slowly across the American landscape. Unlike the wagon train that Samuel Leslie and his family had joined a century before, however, in which the general mood had been one of optimism, the feeling in these caravans was nothing but despair.

In 1830, President Andrew Jackson, Samuel's cousin, signed the Indian Removal Act, which began the process of moving the indigenous people from their ancestral homes in the south to federal land west of the Mississippi River. The land they were to receive was called Indian Territory and included a large portion of the Ozark Mountains. Although the Act eventually led to forced migrations that became known as the "Trail of Tears," it initially allowed for voluntary acquisition of the new land, which many accepted. Among the latter were two brothers, known as Wiley and Owl, who were chiefs in the Cherokee Nation. They both took land high in the Ozarks, and the area where Wiley and his people settled became known as Wiley's Cove.

Years later, another man rode slowly up a rocky road that led higher and higher into the Ozark Mountains. For the young Samuel Leslie, it had the feeling of coming home—home to a place he had never seen. There was something about the rugged, lonely countryside of rolling green meadows and stony outcroppings that reminded him of descriptions he had heard of his ancestral homes in Scotland and Ireland. Spring was in the air. Redbuds were bright with their purple-pink blossoms, the first white petals of dogwoods hung like suspended snowflakes, and a new growth of tender green leaves danced on their branches in the gentle breeze. Maybe it was the feeling of the wind in his hair that gave Samuel a sense of connectedness with the spirit of his lineage—the same feeling that Bartoff had known when the breezes whirled across the moors of Scotland, or that John Leslie had experienced as his ship approached the coast of Ireland, or that his namesake grandfather had felt as he brought his family across the dusty trails of Virginia to a new life in the Carolinas. The winds of Providence had always seemed to beckon his people toward brighter promises beyond each new horizon, and now the sense that his destiny lay within these mountains was almost palpable.

Samuel was the ninth of John and Jane Leslie's ten children and was born two years after they left his grandparents in the Carolinas in 1807 to seek a better life around Barren County in south central Kentucky. It had not been an easy childhood for the young Samuel. He was only two years old when his parents pulled up stakes again and moved to Humphreys County, in the western part of Tennessee. At the tender age of eight, Samuel lost his mother, and his grieving father was faced with the daunting task of raising their large family. In 1825, John received a land grant from the state of Tennessee and he took his children further west over the Natchez Trace to settle in Holly Springs, Carroll County, near the headwaters of Morgan's Creek. Here Samuel would grow to manhood and start his own family.

As Samuel continued up the rocky trail, an orange sun hung low in the sky, bathing the Ozark countryside in a golden glow and casting long shadows down the mountain slopes. The faint pealing of a bell echoed through a distant valley, reminding him that it was Sunday and that people down there were probably heading toward their evening service. And that thought brought a smile to his heart, as he remembered a small country church and another Sunday evening long ago—when he first met Ruth. She was singing in the choir that night, and he remembered thinking that she looked and sounded like an angel. He thought about the first time that he proudly sat with her in church and the first time she let him hold her hand. And he basked in the memory of the time that the two of them stood together in front of family, friends, and God to repeat their wedding vows.

Ruth Harris was a petite, dark-haired beauty and could have won the heart of any man in the county. But her love was for the tall, lanky son of the widower John Leslie. Maybe it was the sincerity she saw in Samuel's hazel eyes, or the dedication to his faith and to making the most of his Providential gifts. Ruth was certain that he was going to do great things in his life, and Samuel was determined not to disappoint her. But opportunities were limited for a young man starting out in Tennessee. With the continued influx of settlers, land was no longer as plentiful as when his father had arrived, and being the ninth of ten children did not put him in line for much of an inheritance. In 1835, at the age of twenty-six, Samuel traveled into Arkansas Territory, which would become the twenty-fifth state of the Union the following year. Something about the land appealed to him, and he had a feeling that here was where he could make his mark in life. Shortly after his return, Samuel and his father had the same talk that John Leslie had had with his father a generation before. John understood the beckoning his son felt, and yet he now recognized the pain that his parents must have known to see their children and grandchildren moving on, probably never to be seen again. For John, that feeling reached its apex on a day in the late winter of 1838, as he watched Samuel and Ruth depart for Arkansas in a covered wagon with their three young children.

The mountains were now settling into the dusk of evening as Samuel neared his destination. The approaching darkness added to his sense of loneliness for his wife and children, whom he had left back in Little Rock. They had made the trip from Tennessee with a few other families that were also moving west, and Samuel's family was staying in their covered wagon with some of their traveling companions. Shortly after arriving in Little Rock, Samuel had gone to the land office to inquire about available property and was told of opportunities in the northwestern highland country of the Ozarks. Before Arkansas had been admitted to statehood, all Indian land titles had been withdrawn by the federal government, and the Native Americans, including those of the Cherokee Nation, were being encouraged to move farther west. Most were peaceful and cooperative and willing to sell their land. Samuel studied a map that was provided in the land office and discovered an area for sale that looked promising about eighty miles north of Little Rock. And so, after a long journey on horseback, he felt that he must be close to his goal, as he caught the scent of wood burning in fireplaces and saw ribbons of smoke rising from chimneys in a nearby cove. Through the fading twilight, he could make out the silhouette of a rough sign and he dismounted to take a closer look. As he read the two words on the sign, Samuel realized that he had indeed reached his destination: WILEY'S COVE.

Ruth's heart sank as she looked out over the scene that was to become their new home. For three exhausting days, her family had been bounced around in their covered wagon, as they climbed ever higher up the rock-strewn road into the hills of the Ozarks. With each turn of the wheels, it seemed that they were leaving civilization farther behind. Now she gazed down on a meager settlement that consisted of nine houses scattered in a cove, with a single dirt street, a small general store, and a post office. But the blood of her pioneer ancestors flowed in her veins, and she hid her disappointment behind a weak smile as she looked up into the enthusiastic eyes of her husband. He had been so excited when he returned to Little Rock to gather his family and take them up to what would become their new home. And, despite her inability to share his enthusiasm, Ruth had complete faith in Samuel's judgment and in his ability to provide for their family. Furthermore, she knew that she had to be strong for her children. Dicy Jane, their oldest at age six, sat between her parents on the front seat of the wagon, seeming to share her mother's opinion of their new home and less inclined to hide it. Behind them on a blanket sat their two younger children, four-year-old Andrew Jackson and three-year-old Mary Ann. In the eyes of young Andy, the land seemed rife with the potential for adventure, as he had listened to his father speak of the opportunities for swimming and fishing. As for little Mary, she was just glad to stop bouncing.

Chief Wiley was no longer a part of the community, having suffered an untimely death a few years earlier, before the government's mandate fulfilled his greatest fear for the future of his people. In memory of the chief, the post office had retained the name Wiley's Cove. Although Samuel's resources were limited, he was able to offer a fair price to an Indian family for a small acreage of land on which he would build a modest, temporary house for his family and begin tilling the soil.

And so the Leslies of Wiley's Cove began the long and arduous process of building a new life for themselves on the American frontier. Like so many pioneers who had gone before them and who would follow, their life would be demanding—laden with back-breaking work, heartaches, fears, and new challenges around every corner. But, with perseverance, ingenuity, and a good measure of faith in Providence, they would not only prosper but would become one of the prominent families in the state, and their little village would become a booming town before the turn of the century.

Within two years of moving to Wiley's Cove, Samuel established a reputation for industry and integrity. He labored from sunrise to sunset, six days each week, building the first home for his family and growing the crops that would provide for their sustenance. And yet he always had time to help a neighbor, whether it was raising a barn, assisting with the calving, or bringing in a harvest before the rain came. But what he may have been most respected for was his steadfast faith. When his father had come to Holly Springs, in Tennessee, he had made friends with several community leaders who were members of the Methodist Church, which had been started by John Wesley in the previous century. John Leslie felt comfortable in this church and soon became an active member, moving his family from their Presbyterian roots to become devout Methodists. One of Samuel's first contributions to their new hometown was to start a small church, built on the teachings of Wesley and his brother, Charles. At first, they met in a home of one of the few congregants, but within a year they had begun construction on a one-room structure that would become the First Methodist Church of Wiley's Cove.

Samuel's reputation spread quickly beyond his little community, and one day he was visited by three prominent citizens of the state who had come up from the capital in Little Rock. Two years earlier, Searcy County, which encompassed Wiley's Cove, had been carved out of Marion County. Samuel learned that the men were state legislators, and he was speechless when they asked if he would consider running for the State Legislature as the representative of Searcy County. At the young age of thirty-one and with no background in legislative matters, he was overwhelmed to receive such an offer. He thanked the men with all the sincerity he could muster and told them that he would send word of his decision within a week. That evening, he and Ruth talked and prayed about what he should do. The modest income would undoubtedly be helpful, but it would require being away from home for a few months each year when the legislature was in session. It may have been his sense of civic responsibility that finally led to his posting a letter to Little Rock, expressing his gratitude and willingness to run for the office. In those days, it was not considered appropriate for a candidate to campaign for himself, so others did that for him. It was most likely his reputation, however, that led to a comfortable victory in the fall. And so it was that the relative newcomer to Arkansas became the Honorable Samuel Leslie of Searcy County.

Samuel was not the only busy person in the family during those early years. Ruth's days also began at or before sunrise and extended well beyond sunset, with cooking, washing, cleaning, sewing, and mending, all with rather primitive implements. From local Indians, for example, she had learned to use the flat, smooth stones that were abundant in the region. In the shallow concavity of a large stone, she would grind corn into meal with a smaller, handheld stone in the mortar and pestle fashion. And she tended to her chores while caring for a bevy of young children whose numbers seemed to grow exponentially. They were barely settled in Wiley's Cove before she gave birth to her fourth child, Eliza, and within little more than a year, the four children were joined by their baby sister, Ruth. Over the course of the next decade, she would give birth to five more children, and all ten would survive infancy and grow to be healthy young adults.

And so, as 1840 was coming to a close, the Leslie family had much to be thankful for, and they never failed to express heartfelt gratitude to the Source of their blessings. But the year ended in a note of sadness when a letter arrived from Tennessee, reporting the death of Samuel's father. His first emotion was more of guilt than of sorrow. Dicy had barely known her grandfather, and Andy and Mary were too young when they had left to have any memory of him. And yet that is the way it was when families were on the move in search of a better life. Samuel's grandfather had left his parents in Ireland to come to the New World, just as John Leslie had left his family in the Carolinas. But, when Samuel had moved his family from Tennessee, he had always hoped that one day his father would come to live with them in Arkansas and see his grandchildren and the life they were making for themselves. Now he didn't even know if his father had lived long enough to receive word that his son had been elected to the State Legislature. He quietly stepped out of the house and looked up into the night sky at the twinkling stars, wondering, as he had many times before, about the mystery of life and death. And then he allowed himself to shed a tear.

Arkansas had been a state for only four years when Samuel took his seat with the other legislators at the State House in Little Rock. He could sense an excitement in the air as his fellow lawmakers contemplated the role they were playing in the history of their state. With each new piece of legislation, they were creating the foundation on which Arkansas would grow in the ages to come. Much of their business was housekeeping. There were still new county boundaries to be defined, local judges and postmasters to be appointed, and roads to be laid out that would one day connect the nascent towns into a thriving state. Although the matter of Indian land had already been settled by the federal government, there was still occasional violence, especially along the western border, and state militias had to be created to protect the new settlers. But the biggest issue of the day, which loomed over virtually every state in the Union—that indeed threatened to explode at any moment and tear the country apart—was slavery.

Samuel was torn by the issue. He was fundamentally opposed to the concept of slavery. The irony in the Declaration of Independence was not lost on him. He knew that not all men in America were at liberty to pursue their happiness. And he would give no comfort to those who used the Bible to justify slavery. To his reading, there was nothing in the scriptures that advocated slavery, but merely acknowledged its existence during Biblical times. And yet there was the practical side. He was, after all, a citizen and representative of a slave state, and the majority of his colleagues in the State House were slave holders, especially those in the southern and eastern regions of the state, where the fertile land supported large cotton plantations. And then there was his cousin and hero, Andrew Jackson—the candidate for whom he had cast his first presidential vote and the man after whom he had named his first son—who owned many slaves on his plantation in Tennessee. The day would soon come when Samuel would also own a few slaves on his farm. But, in his mind, it was not so much the institution of slavery, which he fervently hoped would one day vanish, as it was the right of each state to govern themselves in domestic matters. Like most of his fellow legislators, he bristled at the idea of a remote federal Congress telling them what they could and could not do. And so it was that Samuel Leslie, with considerable reluctance, became a supporter of the pro-slavery faction in his state.

Within four years of their arrival in Wiley's Cove, Samuel had saved enough money to purchase 160 acres of prime farmland, where he built a two-story Southern-style house that would be the family homestead for the next half century. Behind the main house were separate buildings for the kitchen and slave quarters. Samuel was primarily a farmer, and he worked long, hard hours in the fields alongside his slaves to grow a variety of crops. But he was also a businessman. He knew that the prosperity of his family and of the community depended on the growth of the town, and he began a practice in the early days of giving away some of his land to induce other settlers to locate in the Cove. He acquired part ownership in the general store, which he expanded and eventually owned outright, and later invested in a cotton gin and grist mill. He also served as postmaster of their town. Slowly, the sleepy village of Wiley's Cove, in large measure due to the efforts of Samuel Leslie, was beginning to wake up and take its place among the growing towns of Arkansas.

The question of security was becoming an increasing concern. Disgruntled Native Americans continued to stage occasional raids on the outskirts of communities in the western part of the state. An even greater threat was the growing animosity between the pro-slavery and anti-slavery factions among the white settlers. The majority of families in the Ozarks were scratching out a bare-bones existence and many were strongly opposed to slavery. A tension was gradually developing between the two factions, which occasionally erupted in violence. Like his ancestors before him, Samuel was strongly opposed to settling disputes through force of arms. He prayed each day that neighbors could resolve their differences peacefully, and yet he recognized that this was becoming less and less likely. As with his views on slavery, he was finally compelled to see the practical side, which in this case seemed to argue that force was sometimes necessary to achieve peace and to protect his family. And so, again acknowledging his civic and state obligations, he accepted a commission as Lieutenant in the 45th Regiment of the Arkansas Militia. It was not a position he enjoyed or took pride in, but, as with everything else he did, he gave it his full measure of devotion and steadily moved up the ranks, eventually achieving the title of Colonel Samuel Leslie.

As both a military officer and a state legislator, Samuel continued to enjoy the respect and confidence of his colleagues and constituents. It was said that no man had more friends or fewer enemies than he. But the time was coming when men would have to take sides and choose who would be their friends and who would be their enemies. Samuel was re-elected to four more terms in the State Legislature, his fifth victory coming in 1854, and with each new legislative session, he could sense greater tension developing among his fellow statesmen, as their country edged ever closer to armed conflict. A new party, called Republicans, had been formed, and it put up a presidential candidate in 1856. Although the party platform did not call for abolition of slavery, it opposed the expansion of slave states, and the southern states saw this as an unacceptable challenge to their way of life. Samuel had grown weary of the struggles in the State House and opted not to run for a sixth term, feeling that he was going to be needed more back home and in his state militia. And it was not long before his foreboding was realized, when he picked up the local paper on a fall day in 1860 to discover that Abraham Lincoln had been elected president.

During the decade that the winds of impending war were blowing with ever increasing ferocity across the landscape of America, the Leslies of Wiley's Cove were facing their own personal battle. In 1850, Ruth gave birth to their tenth child and fourth son; his parents named him Samuel Evans. He was a quiet, rather serious child and was probably a bit spoiled by his six sisters. But his childhood—indeed his life—was not destined to be easy, as tragedy lurked in many shadows. With each of the last five children that she bore, Ruth seemed to become progressively weaker and she never fully recovered after the arrival of Evans. She did her best to carry on with the demands of a large family, but it was clear that life was ebbing from her, as her weight continuously declined and a racking cough made sleeping almost impossible. The local doctor could offer no cure and warned the family that it was only a matter of time. In the winter of 1859, with Samuel and their ten children around her, Ruth slipped away from them. Evans was about the same age that his father had been when his mother died, and he seemed to take the loss harder than any one else in the family. Samuel was devastated but had little time to mourn, with the responsibility now of such a large family to care for on top of his civic and military obligations. He thanked God that Ruth had been able to hold on until their older children were young adults and able to help with the younger ones and keep the family together. But the family's heartaches were only beginning, as the threat of war loomed ever darker on the horizon.

꩜

South Carolina seceded from the Union even before Lincoln was inaugurated, and other southern states soon followed. Arkansas held off until May 1861, following the Confederates' capture of Fort Sumter and President Lincoln's call for a voluntary Union army. With the Civil War now a reality, Col. Leslie recruited troops for his Arkansas

Militia and trained them for a clandestine operation that he fervently prayed would never materialize. He had received intelligence that a secret organization of Union sympathizers in Searcy County was preparing for an attempted insurrection against the Confederate government. By November, he felt that he could delay no longer and called out six companies of his regiment to break up the organization. By surprising his opponents, many of whom were his neighbors, he was able to quell the insurrection with minimal loss of life on either side and to put seventy-eight members of the opposition in prison. For this achievement, he received recognition by Arkansas Governor Rector. But Samuel took no joy in the victory and only gave thanks that it was accomplished with no greater loss of life. Before Christmas, he dismissed his soldiers so that they could all return to their homes.

Union sentiment remained strong in northern Arkansas, and Samuel was obliged to maintain a ready militia throughout 1862 in order to protect the citizens of Searcy County who were loyal to the Confederacy, which included his family. Since this kept him away from the homestead most of the time, it fell to Andrew, as the oldest son, to run the farm, which was a critical source of food supply for the local Confederate troops. The two middle sons, John and Archibald, both joined the Confederate army as privates, which their father hated but could hardly oppose. John, who was twenty-two years old, was assigned to Company F of the Arkansas Infantry, which was commanded by a Col. Matlock. A large force of Union infantry and cavalry was reported to be marching toward Little Rock, and John's company was among those that were ordered to defend the state capital in what threatened to be a major battle. His brother Archie, who was only seventeen, was assigned to a unit that would be staying in Searcy Country to protect the citizens, much to the relief of his father. At age fifty-four, Samuel could have easily justified staying at home with the local militia, but in 1863 he chose to relinquish his commission of colonel to accept the lower rank of captain in the Confederate army and join Matlock's regiment.

A blistering August sun was bearing down on a line of weary gray-clad soldiers, as they trudged resolutely down a rocky road toward

Little Rock. Leading the platoon was Captain Leslie, who had orders to report to Confederate headquarters at the state capital. The top priority for the Arkansas District of the Confederate army, at that moment, was the defense of their capital, and several thousand troops were gathering around the outskirts of the city. An even larger Federal army was rumored to have crossed the Missouri border and to be heading for a location along the Arkansas River, just a few miles from Little Rock. All the men in Leslie's platoon had seen combat during the past few years and knew the devastation that would be their lot if these two armies clashed. But Samuel had a more personal concern. John had been stationed in the state capital for several months, and his father had been sick with fear for his son's safety. He knew that his own presence would not protect him, but somehow it made him feel better just to know that he would be near him during this treacherous time. And so he was glad to see the silhouette of Little Rock come into view on the horizon.

As they passed one army encampment after another, Samuel could sense not only the heightened state of activity, but also the anxiety in the air. When they arrived at Company F, he gave his men orders to rest before setting up their tents and then went to report to Col. Matlock. The briefing he received was not encouraging. Union cavalry were beginning to cross the Arkansas River, with their infantry close behind them, and a division of Confederate cavalry had been sent out in an attempt to block their passage. It was clear that a major battle was imminent. Samuel asked if he might have a brief visit with his son, which was granted. As he approached their tents, he saw John sitting with some of the other privates. When they saw an officer coming toward them, all the young men jumped to attention and saluted, but father and son could not suppress their emotions as they shook hands, laughed nervously, and then embraced each other.

As the two men stood talking about things back home and the critical situation they were now facing, they looked up to see a chilling sight. The cavalry was returning to the camp—slowly—with their heads down. The most poignant scene was the wounded, who were bringing up the rear. They wore blood-stained bandages that had been hastily wrapped around their heads, over an eye, or where so recently an arm or leg had been. Some were able to stay on their horses, while others walked with help, having had their horse shot out from under them; still others rode in wagons, clinging to life. And yet these were the fortunate ones. Many of their comrades had been left behind—lifeless bodies strewn across the field of battle. Samuel turned his head so that his son would not see the tears in his eyes. He knew this meant that their cavalry had failed to block the advance of the Federal army, which would soon be forming battle lines around Little Rock. He blotted his eyes and faced his son with a look of tenderness and resolve. They silently embraced, both praying that it would not be for the last time.

The commander of the Confederate army in the Arkansas District was Major General Sterling Price. He had been given an exaggerated report regarding the size of the advancing Union forces and was more concerned about saving his army than holding the capital. It had not been long since his fellow officer, General Pemberton, had been trapped in a similar situation at Vicksburg, and he vowed not to let this happen in Little Rock. He promptly ordered an immediate evacuation of the capital, and the Confederate army began a hasty but orderly retreat toward the south, leaving the Arkansas capital in the hands of the Union. And so Samuel and John were spared the horrors of a major encounter that day and lived to fight other battles.

Company F was ordered to Arkadelphia, a small town about seventy miles southwest of Little Rock, where they set up camp and waited for what the war would bring next. Days dragged into weeks as the boredom of camp life set in, broken only by drills and occasional patrols. As the last leaves of autumn drifted to the ground, it became apparent that this would be their winter camp, and it was about then that Samuel began to fear that something was wrong. For several days, a sense of weakness and mild nausea had been growing progressively worse. Then one night he awoke sometime in the dark predawn to discover that his whole body was chilled and that he could not control his shaking, despite being soaked with perspiration. He had a splitting headache and every muscle in his body seemed to ache. He lay on his cot, waiting for the dawn and hoping that his symptoms would pass. But, when the bugle announced morning muster and he attempted to get up, he collapsed on the floor of his tent—and that was where they found him. He was delirious by the time he was discovered by his orderly and, when the company doctor arrived, he pronounced Captain Leslie to have been stricken with malaria.

American medicine during the Civil War was just emerging from the middle ages of medical history. Ether and nitrous oxide were being used for general anesthesia, which was a Godsend for those requiring amputations or other surgery. But the germ theory of disease and the importance of antisepsis in treating wounds were yet to be understood. The water supply in many camps was contaminated by nearby latrines and infested with disease-bearing insects. Surgeons did not routinely wash their hands between operations or use clean instruments or dressings. As a result, there were numerous intractable camp illnesses including diarrhea, dysentery, typhoid, and malaria, and gangrene was a common sequel of wound treatment. Of the estimated 620,000 deaths in the war, twice as many soldiers died of disease as of battle wounds. And Samuel Leslie had now joined the countless thousands whose personal battle in the Civil War would be more with germs than steel.

For a month he lay in the makeshift camp hospital on the precipice of death, fluctuating in and out of lucidity. John was allowed to minister to his father's needs whenever his unit was not on patrol, and he did his best to comfort him both physically and spiritually. It frustrated him that medical science had so little to offer, and he even questioned what value religion, in its present form, provided the sick and dying soldiers. It may have been those thoughts while at his father's bedside, during some of his darkest hours, that would one day lead John to his choice of professions.

Christmas Day in the winter camp that year was a somber time for all the homesick soldiers. The pensive strains of carols could be heard around some of the campfires, and well wishes echoed across the fields as comrades tried to bolster each other's spirits. John spent the day at his father's side. A package had arrived earlier from the family back in Wiley's Cove. It contained a pound of coffee—a prized commodity in those days—and a tin of cookies, which had grown hard with time, but still had the taste of home. Most welcomed, however, were the personal greetings from each of their loved ones. John read them aloud to Samuel several times. Then he opened his Bible and read the old familiar passages from the prophet Isaiah and the gospel of Luke. After a reverent silence, as the two men reflected on the beauty of the words and thought about home, John began singing one of his father's favorite Christmas carols in a soft voice, and Samuel attempted to join in. For both of them, it was the saddest, loneliest Christmas they had ever known, and yet in its own way it was the most beautiful.

With the first breath of spring in the air, Samuel began to feel his strength returning. He had always hoped that he would eventually be able to resume his military duties, but the doctor informed him that that was not possible. He would need many more months of rest if he ever hoped to regain his full health. And so his time in the army came to an end, and he began making preparations to return home. He bid an emotional farewell to his fellow officers and the men in his platoon and then spent his last evening in camp with John. They read a few passages from their Bibles, prayed together, and then embraced in a tearful farewell.

Samuel rode home in a wagon driven by a one-armed soldier and accompanied by two escorts on horseback. With the Union army occupying Little Rock and sending patrols out into the surrounding countryside, it was a treacherous journey, and all four men wore civilian clothes to minimize their risk. But Samuel's thoughts tended less toward his safety than to his sense of guilt for deserting his companions and especially for leaving his son in harm's way. John would be in his thoughts and prayers constantly until he too came home. And yet, as the wagon pulled into Wiley's Cove, Samuel had to admit that he was thrilled to be there. Andrew had done a good job of keeping the farm running. Dicy had married just before her father left, and she and her husband, John Boyd, were helping Andrew run the farm. The other five daughters, Mary, Eliza, Ruth, Nancy, and Ann, were also doing their part in the house and in the fields, as well as contributing to the local war effort. Evans was now fourteen and capable of putting in the day's work of a man, although his heart was bent on joining the Confederate army and wearing a uniform like his brother Archie.

Of all his children, it was probably Archie that Samuel was happiest to see. Although Archie's position in the army was less dangerous than John's, Samuel had prayed no less fervently for his safety. He was so proud to see how handsome Archie looked in his uniform and how he carried himself with such confidence and dignity. Since his unit was stationed in Searcy County, he was able to come home frequently and he spent much of that time at his father's bedside, telling him about his latest military experiences—which he had to admit were rather dull—and talking about his plans when the war was over. He was considering many careers, but was leaning most strongly toward the ministry. That made Samuel especially pleased, as he had once considered the same direction for his own life, and it made him realize how much the two of them had in common. One evening, just before Archie was scheduled to return to his platoon, Samuel told his son how much he loved him and how proud he was of him and how optimistic he was for his bright future. To his dying day, Samuel would always thank God that he had spoken those words to Archie that night, because they were to be the last words that he would ever say to his son.

Wiley's Cove had been spared any major battles during the Civil War, the closest having been near the town of Marshall, a few miles to the north. But the citizens of the town and surrounding area remained deeply divided between their loyalty to the Union and to the Confederacy. There were those who would not think twice about killing a neighbor who they considered to be an enemy. Some, known as "bushwhackers," would lie in wait with their rifle to ambush and kill unsuspecting victims. Early in the morning, after Archie had spent the evening with his father, he was riding back to camp when a bullet came from an unseen assailant somewhere in the thick forest and went through his skull. When his comrades found him later that morning, they concluded that death must have come instantly.

That evening, as the sun was beginning to set, the Leslie family was gathered in Samuel's bedroom, mourning together in stunned silence. And, as they sat there in the stillness, amid tears and embraces, a most unexpected thing happened. From just outside the bedroom window, they heard the gentle strains of soft, mournful music. Andrew rose, walked over to the window and looked out to see all their family of slaves standing below him with bowed heads. The men and boys were holding their hats in front of them, and the women and little girls were raising their hands with palms toward heaven. They were singing a hymn that Samuel and his family had heard them sing many times in their prayer meetings, "Steal away, steal away home." Andrew turned and looked at his father, and Samuel knew what it was without a spoken word. He struggled to get out of bed and made his way to the front door and out onto the porch and over to the side where his slaves were still singing. Samuel had always felt the guilt of being a slave owner, and in that moment he thought again how much we are all like brothers. He knew that he would find it difficult to speak, being so overwhelmed with emotions, but he was finally able to whisper, "Thank you."

The war finally and mercifully ended, and the fortunate families were reunited with their loved ones. John Leslie was among those who returned home, despite having fought in several skirmishes in Arkansas up to the end of the war. For his valor and leadership, he was promoted to the rank of an officer and came home to Wiley's Cove as Major Leslie. However, that now had little significance, since the Confederacy no longer existed, and the South was bracing for the aftermath of the war. The new president, Andrew Johnson, claimed to be doing his best to fulfill the dream of Abraham Lincoln for a charitable reconciliation. But Johnson was no match for the strong Congress, which had other ideas about what they called Reconstruction. It is hard to know what is truly in the mind of another person. Some of the Congressmen undoubtedly believed that their plan was in the best interest of the African Americans for whose freedom they had so diligently labored, but others seemed to be driven more by a vitriolic sense of retribution, and still others appeared to be interested only in personal gain. Whatever the motivations may have been, the years that followed would impose unimaginable tribulations on both the white and Black people of the South and would exacerbate racial tensions that would last for the next century and beyond.

On the morning that he received confirmation that the war was truly over and that the Emancipation Proclamation would become the law of the land, Samuel met on the front lawn with his slaves. The leader of the small family of blacks was a white-haired gentleman by the name of Isaiah. He and Samuel were about the same age, and over the years the two men had developed a friendship of sorts. When they were all settled on the lawn in quiet anticipation of what they might hear, Samuel began.

"Well, Isaiah, looks like you and your folks are free now, and you can leave whenever you wish. And you will go with my blessings."

There was a long silence, as the former slaves looked at each other and then toward Isaiah. Their expressions conveyed more uncertainty and fear than joy, and Isaiah explained their feelings.

"Thank you, suh. But where would we go? Ain't no place safe fo' us colored folk in these parts, and how would we find work?"

Samuel had anticipated this response and had been giving it serious consideration. His conscience had never given him peace since acquiring slaves, and he felt that he had an obligation to them.

"Well, Isaiah," he began slowly, "you are always welcome to stay here. You can keep your homes and improve them as you wish. We will always need your help in the fields and in the house, and I will pay each of you wages for your work. And you can have some plots of ground to grow food for your family. And, of course, you can always leave whenever you wish."

As he was completing his words, those sitting on the lawn looked at each other and nodded with an unspoken agreement that this is what they wanted. And so the country's awful conflict came to an end and, while much of the South continued to smolder in hatred and confusion, a feeling of hope for a better future was taking root in at least one small community high in the Ozarks.

The final decades of the nineteenth century saw growth and prosperity for the Leslie family and for their town of Wiley's Cove. The downtown area now had two dirt streets, Main and Oak, at right angles to each other, and boasted four stores. Andrew had become a leading citizen of the community and built a large home on the corner of the two streets for his wife, Sara, and their two children. John and his wife, Elizabeth, purchased a large farm just outside of Marshall, where they began raising their six children. He became a doctor and a Baptist minister, career choices that may have been influenced by memories of those dark hours during the war when he had cared for his sick father. And, like his father, John also served in the Arkansas state legislature. Evans Leslie started a small farm on the outskirts of Wiley's Cove for his wife, Callie, and their three children.

But life was not without heartaches for the Leslie family. Samuel's two oldest daughters, Dicy and Mary, died during the war and were buried beside each other in the city cemetery. They left behind nine children between them, and the two youngest came to live with Samuel. Ruth lost her husband, and she and her only child, Mollie, also moved back to the family homestead. Andrew's wife, Sara, died at a young age, and he married her sister, Melinda, who gave birth to ten more children. John also lost his wife, Elizabeth, leaving him with six young children, and he later married Martha, who brought seven more children into their family. Eliza had four children and Ann had ten, although most of Ann's died in childhood. Only Nancy never married. And so Samuel was surrounded by a host of children, grandchildren, and eventually great-grandchildren, and although he never fully recovered from the grief of each loss, he never failed to pray daily for their souls and to thank God for those who were still with him.

By the turn of the century, the sleepy village of a few homes that Samuel had first encountered would grow into a thriving community of over 4,000 citizens. Virgin growths of hardwood timber, which stretched in all directions from Wiley's Cove, would eventually lead to a booming woodworking industry. Much of the local oak was used to make barrels, and the town became known as the "Barrel Capital of the World." In addition, the town would eventually boast a cigar factory, carding mill, broom factory, tin shop, ice and light plant, brick kiln, and box-making plant. Trains would one day pull into a handsome stone station, and the five hotels would barely be able to accommodate all the travelers. Although Samuel would not live to see all of these advances, many of which occurred in the first two decades of the twentieth century, it was clear that the town in his time was well on its way to bigger and better things. And it was also clear that one man, more than any other, was responsible for this progress.

And so, on a warm summer day in 1886, under a clear blue sky, virtually every citizen of Wiley's Cove gathered on the street near the post office to witness what might well be the most important moment in the town's history. A wooden platform, festooned in red, white, and blue bunting, had been erected, and on it sat Samuel Leslie and his sons, Andrew and John. For many years, there had been discussion about changing the name of the post office and, thereby, the name of the town. Andrew, with the help of John in the state legislature, had been able to pass a bill that would legally sanction that change.

As a hush fell over the crowd, Andrew rose and stepped up to the podium. He recounted the history of their town, how it had been only a few homes when the first white settlers came in the 1830s, and how his father had stimulated its growth by giving away his own land to new settlers. He told of how his father had represented them in the state legislature and how he had protected them in both the Arkansas militia and the Confederate army and had served as their postmaster before and after the war. The people listened and nodded their heads toward each other, as though to agree that the change which was about to be announced was most appropriate. And so it was on that day that Wiley's Cove officially became Leslie, Arkansas.

Standing back in the crowd of people that morning was a twelve-year-old boy, who listened with pride to the accolades being bestowed upon his grandfather. His only regret was that his father could not be on the platform with the other men of his family. Nevertheless, looking at his grandfather, sitting so tall and dignified with his silky white hair and firm but gentle demeanor, gave him a great sense of Providence to be a part of such a distinguished and respected family. He couldn't help but wonder if he would ever be able to live up to the standards of his elders and one day bring credit to his family. But there was one thing he knew for certain, as he stood there among his family and friends: he would always be blessed with a host of good, God-fearing people to support him in whatever he would attempt to accomplish in his life.

CHAPTER 5

Indian Territory

1884–1893

"COME ALONG NOW, CHILDREN. It's time we were headin' home."

Bruce Leslie didn't seem to hear his mother. His mind was somewhere off in deep thought, which was becoming an increasingly common trait for him. It was not that he was disrespectful to his mother. On the contrary, he had always been extremely respectful to all his elders. But, more and more, he seemed to be at the mercy of an active mind that could carry him away into such deep thought that he could be totally oblivious to everything around him. And at that moment his mind was still on the honor that had just been bestowed on his grandfather. But, more than that, he was thinking about his father.

He was tall for his age and rather slender. "Lanky" was how some described him. During the past two years, he had taken on the work of a grown man, which gave him the appearance of maturity beyond his age. It was generally agreed that he most closely favored his grandfather, Samuel Leslie, an observation that would become increasingly apparent as he grew to manhood. Even now, his hazel eyes seemed to reflect his grandfather's mixture of thoughtfulness and good humor—a frequent twinkle that revealed his joy for life. But now those eyes seemed to express only a pensive sadness.

Bruce was stirred from his reverie by the gentle touch of a hand in his. He turned and gazed into his mother's eyes and gave her a warm smile. And, with a self-conscious chuckle, he looked over and smiled at his little sister. Both women loved his smile. It was broad and sincere, although usually with his lips tightly pursed. But none of them really felt like smiling at that moment, as they stood on the dusty street and watched the last of the town folks drifting back to their shops and homes. The wooden platform, still festooned in its red, white, and blue bunting, was empty now, which added to the sense of emptiness that the three of them were feeling. But their mother took both of them by the hand and, with her best effort at a cheery smile, began walking them home.

Their mother's maiden name was California Jamima Hatchett, and she was known as Callie when she met Evans Leslie and became his wife in the early 1870s. As she walked home between her two children, she marveled at how large and strong Bruce's hands had become in his short twelve years of life. And her thoughts drifted back to a spring day when that same hand had grasped hers for the first time and was barely large enough to wrap around her little finger.

Samuel Brewster Leslie was born on April 6, 1874, in the town that was now named for his grandfather. It was a day that Callie would always consider to be one of the most blessed of her life. His smile was there from the beginning, and Callie, with a typical mother's loving pride, was convinced that no child could have been more perfect as he grew from infancy to boyhood. He was neither her first child nor her last. His brother, Green Evans, known as Eb, was two years older, and his sister, Floy Tilden, a year younger. But there was something about the relationship between Bruce and his mother that would bind them from his birth until her final day.

As children, Eb, Bruce, and Floy were the best of friends and took full advantage of all the wonders that their home in the Ozarks had to offer young people. They attended the same one-room school, although sessions were only for three months of the year, which gave them considerable time for more pleasurable activities. When the day's chores were done, they loved to roam the seemingly endless hills and woods around their home. And there were the clear and swiftly flowing streams, where countless hours were spent on hot summer days swimming in the deliciously cold water, or relaxing on the banks with their fishing poles extended out over the stream.

There was an abundance of delicacies in the woods to grace their dinner table. In the early spring, little green berries would begin to appear on the bushes, which would soon ripen into juicy red strawberries, tangy blueberries, and succulent blackberries, the latter of which Callie would incorporate into her delicious cobblers, one of Bruce's favorites throughout his life. In the fall, the trees would begin to yield their bounty of pecans, walnuts, and chestnuts, which the children would gather in anticipation of the treats their mother would make from them to enjoy on cold winter days. Another autumn pleasure was the grapes that hung down in clusters from vines in the trees, filling the woods with a luscious fragrance and their bellies with wonderful-tasting fruit and juice.

As Eb and Bruce grew older, they were allowed to go hunting with their father. Neither hunting nor fishing was looked upon by Evans as idle sport, but as an important part of their daily life in order to put food on their table. And yet, tramping through the woods beside their father and being taught to carry and shoot a rifle were among childhood's greatest joys for the two brothers. For all three of the Leslie children, those early halcyon years would forever live in their memories as the most beautiful of times. They felt secure and loved in their tightly knit little family, and life was good. But then, in one tragic moment, it all came tumbling down.

As the youngest of Samuel Leslie's ten children, Evans always seemed to struggle in the shadows of his three brothers. Andrew had become a highly successful businessman and one of the most respected citizens in the community. After Wiley's Cove became Leslie, Arkansas, he succeeded his father as the town's postmaster. John was probably the most successful of the brothers, having served in the Confederate army and now a practicing physician as well as a Baptist minister. In time, he would also follow in his father's footsteps by being elected to the state legislature. And then there was Archie. What can you say about a brother who gave his life to protect his family and friends? His death had given him a special spot in the hearts of all the Leslies that none could ever replace.

This is not to say that Bruce's father, Evans, was without his own virtues. He was a loving husband and father, who worked tirelessly to provide for his family. But he was never able to give them the same standard of living that his kin enjoyed. They had a modest house on a small farm near the outskirts of town. The land was barely sufficient to grow enough crops and raise a few chickens to feed the family. Evans also managed the general store in town, which was their only source of steady income, although the narrow profit margin typically yielded just enough for their bare necessities. But the children never believed that they were poor, and they felt secure in the love of their family.

Of his two parents, Bruce was closest to his mother. She was the one he could confide in, who cared for him when he was sick, who helped him with his homework, who praised him for his achievements. She was the one who read to him each night and said his prayers with him before tucking him in. And she was the one who got her children up on Sunday mornings and dressed them and took them to church. Bruce's relationship with his father was more formal. From him, he learned to hunt and fish and grow things in the fields. But there was never the same intimacy between them as with his mother. This may have been in part because Evans was away so much of the time, struggling to make ends meet for his family. Even on Sunday mornings, there was always something that needed to be done on the farm, and he only rarely attended church with his family. While Bruce's feeling for his mother was one of abiding affection, the emotion he felt for his father was more of respect and gratitude. But then the day came when Bruce would realize how much he truly loved his father.

It was in the fall of 1884, when Bruce was ten, that his father announced he had a business venture that would not only give his family the best Christmas yet, but would provide for their comfort throughout the coming winter. He had met two men who were hunters and who knew where game was plentiful in nearby Benton County. They were going there for a few weeks and would bring back enough meat not only to feed the family through the winter but also to sell in the general store for a handsome profit. Callie and the children would have to manage the farm and the store while he was away.

And so, on a crisp autumn morning, with the two men waiting outside on their horses, Evans said goodbye to his family. He kissed his wife on the cheek and pecked Floy on the top of her head. Then he shook hands with his two sons, admonishing them to protect the women while he was away. Callie stood with her children in the doorway of their home, watching the three men ride off on their horses, their rifles slung over their backs. None of them could have known how fateful that moment was in their lives.

A week had passed when Callie heard a horse galloping at top speed up the road toward their home. She looked out the window to see one of her husband's fellow hunters riding up breathlessly. He jumped down, met her at the front door, and announced that there had been an accident. Evans had gone into some brush to flush out the game, when one of his companions mistook the movement for an animal and fired, hitting Evans. They did not think that it was a life-threatening wound, but he would need time for nursing and recovery. At the moment, he was resting in the cabin they had rented for their hunting trip and was being attended by a local doctor. Evans had indicated that he wanted to come home as soon as possible to recuperate, and the hunter offered to guide Callie to her husband so that she could help bring him home.

Callie immediately went into action. She told Eb to mind the store and Floy to take care of the house, while she and Bruce would take the family wagon to bring their father home. Early the next morning, they headed out, with the hunter leading the way. The air was tense with emotions, but Bruce and his mother tried to console each other with reminders of how blessed they were that the wound had not been fatal. Sadly, they knew only half of the story.

It was true that the gunshot wound Evans suffered should not have threatened his life, since the bullet lodged in his right shoulder away from his lungs and any major blood vessels. But when the doctor arrived he inserted his unwashed finger into the wound to locate the bullet. Although the germ theory was gaining traction in England and Europe, American doctors were still strangely indifferent to one of the most important advances in medical history. The germs that the doctor introduced into the bullet wound spread through Evans's bloodstream, creating an overwhelming infection that no treatment of that day could overcome.

When Callie and Bruce entered the one-room cabin, they found Evans lying in feverish perspiration and nearly delirious. Both were shocked and perplexed to find him in this condition. A harried, disconsolate doctor sat in a straight wooden chair beside his patient. His body language seemed to express the frustration of watching yet another patient slip from his grasp. He rose slowly from his chair and shuffled toward the new arrivals. After brief introductions, he proceeded to explain the situation with the best professionalism and compassion that he could muster.

"Mrs. Leslie, your husband is very ill. The bullet that entered his body is releasing poison into his system." While this was not factual, it was the generally accepted theory among the local medical community of the time. "The poison has now spread throughout his body, and his body is doing all it can to fight it off. Within the next few days or weeks, we will know if his body is strong enough to win the battle or...."

His words trailed off, as though he could not bring himself to complete the sentence, even though he had said it so many times before. He explained that the most they could do was to make Evans as comfortable as possible, and he expressed his pleasure that the family was there to help with that. Callie was a woman of pioneer stock who had learned to face every form of hardship with fortitude and resourcefulness. There were no tears or distress, only a calm acceptance of the situation and a request for more details as to how best to care for her husband. Bruce listened quietly but carefully to the conversation, storing up impressions and memories that would return to him many times in the years to come.

Callie stayed up with Evans the entire night following their arrival. She cooled his feverish brow with a wet cloth and helped him take sips of water through his parched lips. It seemed to give him strength, or maybe it was just her presence. In any case, he became more alert and expressed his gratitude and pleasure to have her by his side. She read to him from her Bible and prayed with him. She held his hand, as he drifted off to sleep, and then she continued to pray silently.

When the first shafts of morning light filtered through the cabin window, Callie was still sitting beside her husband, holding his hand, her Bible in her lap. Bruce had slept on a blanket in a corner of the cabin, and the two hunting companions had slept outside, pledging to stay for as long as they were needed. The doctor had gone home but promised that he would return each day to check on his patient. As daylight filled the room, Bruce awoke and came to his mother's side. He convinced her to refresh herself, eat a bite, and then lie down and get some sleep, while he sat with his father. And that was the way each day would go—Bruce sitting with his father during much of the daylight hours and Callie with him throughout the night, although she slept very little during the day.

On the third day, Andrew and John arrived in Andrew's buckboard, having been notified by one of the hunters that their brother's situation was grave. John had brought his doctor's bag, with his instruments and medications, hoping he might be able to offer something more than was being done. But, when he saw Evans's condition, he sadly realized that it was not so much his doctor's hat that his brother needed as his minister's hat. He took Callie and Bruce aside and told them that they should prepare for the worst.

Despite the foreboding prognosis, Callie maintained her outward appearance of strength and continued to minister to her husband almost every waking moment. As Bruce sat by his father's side each day, he began to feel a closeness to him that he had never experienced before. Evans told his son how proud he was of him and how confident he was that Bruce would do great things in his life and be just as distinguished as any of his Leslie relatives.

One day, when it was clear that he would not last much longer, Evans feebly asked his son to bring him his saddlebag and take a book from it. When Bruce did so, he was surprised to find that it was a Bible, one that had obviously seen a great deal of use. Evans explained that it had been given to him by his father. With a painful attempt at a jocular smile, he suggested that his father probably thought he needed it more than his other children. He admitted that he had neglected it over the years, but something had caused him to pack it in his saddlebag when he left on his fateful hunting trip. He told Bruce that he wanted him to have it, and, as father and son placed their hands on the Bible, they looked deeply into each other's eyes, possibly for the first time.

As Bruce opened the Bible to the family record page, he found that it contained many signatures. Some were so old and faded that he could not make them out with certainty. But four were clearly visible:

Samuel Leslie, b. 1735 County Antrim, Ireland

John Leslie, b. 1765 Waxhaw, The Carolinas

Samuel Leslie, b. 1809 Barren County, Kentucky

Samuel Evans Leslie, b. 1850 Wiley's Cove, Arkansas

Evans's condition began to deteriorate precipitously just after the poignant encounter with his son. It was as though he had now done all he could to fulfill his earthly aspirations and was ready to face whatever lay ahead. Callie was now staying at his side virtually around the clock, with little or no sleep. Andrew had gone back home to attend to business, but John stayed behind to do whatever he could for his younger brother and his family. The sun was disappearing behind the distant hills, and Bruce was sitting with his uncle and the two hunters outside the cabin, when Callie came to the door and told him that his father was asking for him. As he entered the cabin, he had to stop for a moment and brace himself against the putrid smell in the room that came from the unchecked infection. It was one of the many stenches of disease and death that Bruce would come to recognize all too well in the years ahead.

As he approached the bed, Bruce realized that his father had fallen back into an unconscious state, although his labored breathing assured him that he was still alive. He sat down beside him, and his thoughts began to drift. He remembered the times they had sat together on the bank of a stream with their fishing poles extended over the clear water, and those days when they walked side by side through the dense forests with their rifles slung over their shoulders. He remembered the kindness and love his father had shown to his family, in his own way. But he also remembered wondering why he didn't go to church with the family, which he knew made his mother sad. Maybe he had found God in other ways—in the beauty of a flowing stream or the stillness of the primal forest. The recent gift of the Bible only added to his quandary, but he had to conclude that he would never fully know what was in his father's heart.

As he was mulling over all these thoughts, he saw his father stir. He partially opened his bloodshot eyes and reached out with a trembling, sweaty hand to his son. Bruce could see that he wanted to say something to him, but the words were coming hard and he could barely whisper. Bruce leaned closer to hear and could just make out his hoarse words.

"Take your mother...to church."

They were the last words that Samuel Evans Leslie ever spoke. When his wife came back into the room, after giving father and son a respectful time together, she found Bruce by his father's side with tears flowing down his cheeks and her husband lying silent. She asked John to come in, and he checked for his brother's breathing and pulse and then slowly pulled the sheet over his face. For the first time, Callie allowed herself to cry. She sat in the corner with her ten-year-old son, and the two of them held hands and cried for a long time. Then she lay down and slept for the first time in days.

The following morning, at the first crack of dawn, the family prepared to take Evans's body home. The hunters had hastily built a pine wood coffin the night before, and they helped John gently place the body in it and then load it on the wagon. They draped a black sheet over it, and Bruce and his uncle put on black arm bands and took their seats in the front of the wagon. Callie wore a black dress and veil that John had purchased for her in the nearby town, and she sat in the back on a blanket beside the coffin. The two hunters stayed behind and, after expressing their regrets and condolences, stood respectfully as the wagon slowly disappeared down the dusty road.

The appearance of the wagon made it clear that this was a funeral cortege, and farmers in their fields would stop their work, remove their straw hats, and stand silently until it had passed. No words were spoken on the wagon, and Bruce soon drifted into his deep thoughts. It was getting on toward evening when he was suddenly roused from his daydreaming by a gentle breeze. It had been a warm, dry day, and the coolness of the breeze was not only refreshing but somehow comforting. And then he felt a gentle hand on his shoulder. Assuming that it was his mother, he turned to give her a smile, but saw that she was still back beside the coffin and sound asleep. He turned to his uncle, but his eyes were fixed straight ahead with both hands on the reins. He looked around to see if there was anyone else, but they were all alone. He concluded that it must have been his imagination, probably helped by the wind that was getting stronger. And yet he had the strange feeling that they were not entirely alone.

As they neared the family farm, there was one more hill to go around, but Bruce knew a shortcut over the hill and asked if he might get out and walk the rest of the way. His mother and uncle suspected that he needed time alone before returning to the house, and they were pleased to grant his request. The Bible had been sitting on the seat beside Bruce, and his uncle handed it to him as he stepped down from the wagon. He gave his mother a warm smile and then turned and started up toward the wooded trail.

The wind was rustling the leaves of the trees overhead as Bruce ventured deeper into the forest. He felt it swirling around his head and, at times, he looked to see if there was anyone else on the trail. The feeling that he was not alone had stayed with him from the wagon to the woods, and he finally stopped to look around and listen to the wind and feel its gentle touch. A large, smooth stone beckoned him to sit for a while. Looking down at the Bible in his hands, he opened it and found himself in the book of John. His eyes were drawn to a verse that someone had underlined in faint pencil: *"The wind bloweth where it listeth, and thou hearest the sound thereof, but canst not tell whence it cometh, and whither it goeth: so is every one that is born of the Spirit."*

Even at the tender age of 10, Bruce could not help but wonder about the irony of discovering the passage as he sat alone with the wind blowing about him. In the years to come, he would ponder many more mysteries of his life. At the moment, however, he began to wonder who it was that might have underlined the passage. Was it his grandfather or one of the more distant relatives whose names were inscribed in the book? Whoever it was, he believed that he was beginning to understand why he did not feel alone, even on this deserted path. His heritage of courageous, God-fearing people who had gone before him was a blessing that would strengthen and guide him in whatever lay ahead on his road of life. In the years to come, Bruce would look back on that moment as a major turning point in his life.

Not long after their father's funeral, Eb moved to Texas to live with relatives, leaving Bruce as the "man of the family." Financial problems began almost immediately for Callie and her two remaining children. Andrew informed her that the general store did not belong to her family, but that Evans had only managed it. Since he felt that neither she nor her children were in a position to run it, Andrew took over the responsibility. He promised her that she would share in the profits, although it seemed that the profit margin was never sufficient for any income to trickle down to her family. So Bruce had to do whatever he could to help his mother and sister keep their little family afloat. While Floy assisted with chores in the house, he worked beside his mother in the field and took any odd jobs that came his way. He worked with his uncles to plant their crops in the spring and harvest them in the fall. He also worked for neighboring farmers in their corn fields and cotton fields. He cut wood, split rails for fences, and found part-time employment in a nearby cotton gin and a grist mill. But, come Sundays, he would always set aside his work and accompany his mother and sister to church.

His education had to be put on hold, although he was determined that this would be only a temporary situation, since he had a burning ambition to improve his mind and one day find a noble calling that would be a credit to his heritage. In addition to his Bible, he read everything that he could get his hands on. One of the professions that he considered at an early age was teaching, and he became friendly with the local schoolmarm, who helped him with his penmanship in the Spencerian style of the day. He also saved every penny he could in order to one day further his education. His habit of saving money, developed at such a young age, was one of the traits that would stay with him throughout his life. In later years, he preferred to call it "fiduciary prudence," although most people just said he was "frugal." No one would ever accuse him of being stingy, however, as he was always the first to share his blessings with those in need. In any case, the pennies added up and by the age of fifteen he had saved enough money to take a one-year course at nearby Valley Springs Academy, which qualified him to try his hand at teaching.

Bruce's first teaching assignment was in the small settlement of Owl's Cove, which had been named for Chief Wiley's brother, Owl, and was just a few miles from Leslie. He was now a member of the salaried workforce, receiving the respectable income of $25 a month. However, this was not quite enough to live on, and he "boarded around" by rotating among the homes of his pupils, where he received free room and board.

While Bruce was living and working in Owl's Cove, his mother met a man by the name of David Marrs, a widower living in Madison County in the town of St. Paul on the White River about thirty-six miles up from Fayetteville. Callie married David that same year and moved to St. Paul. Bruce had been missing his mother, and now the separation from her was even greater, so he elected to leave his present situation and seek a teaching position in St. Paul. First, however, he had to take an examination in order to obtain a teaching license in Madison County. He returned to Leslie, where Floy was still living, and the two of them rode the old family mule to the town of Hinesville, about 21 miles from St. Paul, where they both took and passed the teacher's examination. Then they moved to St. Paul to be with their mother and step-father.

Bruce taught school for two terms in St. Paul. He found teaching to be stimulating and rewarding, and he seemed to have an aptitude for it. He was instantly popular with his students, especially with the girls, who shyly admired their handsome young teacher. But, while he enjoyed and appreciated the privilege of enriching young minds, it was clear that the monetary rewards of teaching were limited, and Bruce began to wonder if his calling might lie elsewhere.

His frugality continued to serve him well, and he saved enough from his teacher's salary to enter Arkadelphia Practical Business College in the town where his grandfather and uncle had been stationed during the War. Admission to the college included a much-needed $75 scholarship, the certificate of which indicated that S. B. Leslie was entitled "to a full Diploma Business Course of instructions... embracing Book-keeping, Banking, Practical Penmanship, Business Arithmetic...etc." The school was generous with the necessary study materials, stating only that "Students are required to furnish their own writing paper to practice on." However, they also had a strict disciplinary code, including the statement that "This Scholarship is issued and accepted with the understanding that it will be forfeited if the holder is absent without permission." Bruce was meticulously punctual in his attendance and earnestly diligent in his studies, and he graduated with honors in 1893.

Now, as a man of letters, Bruce sought an opportunity to apply his newly acquired business skills. This led him to the headquarters of the Bently & Cobb Nursery, which was advertising for a salesman. The company sold fruit trees and was looking for a representative to extend their sales west of Arkansas into Indian Territory. For a nineteen-year-old who had never ventured far beyond northwest Arkansas, this seemed like another world, and his mother worried about his safety among all those Indians.

"There ain't really much to worry about, Mr. Leslie," Simon Cobb said, as he leaned back in his swivel oak chair and blew a cloud of cigar smoke toward the ceiling. "The Indians in those parts are pretty well settled and civilized by now, especially in the Creek Nation, which would be your sales district."

Bruce wasn't altogether convinced. "I've heard stories about divisions among the Creeks that have led to violence and murder," he said.

"Oh well, that was a long time ago," Cobb responded, "back when the government was forcing the Creeks out of their eastern land. An upper division of mostly full-blood Creeks—Red Sticks, I think they were called—resisted and took revenge on their brothers to the south. Many of the lower Creeks had married into Scottish families in Georgia and were half-bloods. They tried to make the most of the white man's offers, which angered the Red Sticks. But, like I say, that was a long time ago. Most of the full-bloods keep pretty much to themselves, but the half-bloods have become quite successful farmers. And white settlers are also movin' into the area, so we think it's gonna be a good market for our trees."

Bruce remained silent and appeared thoughtful and still unconvinced, and Cobb began to fear that he was losing his potential salesman.

"Mr. Leslie," he said, "we are prepared to offer you a base salary of $50 a month plus a bonus of 15¢ for every tree you sell. With the district that you'll be going into, we believe there is the potential for a handsome profit."

Bruce was listening more intently now. He did some quick calculations in his head and realized that this was indeed a chance to earn enough money to fund whatever future opportunities might come his way.

"Well, sir, that is a very generous offer," he said with a smile. And then, after another moment of thought, he added, "And I am pleased to accept it."

Cobb's concerned countenance suddenly turned into a big, relieved smile, as he reached across the desk, thrust out his beefy hand and shook that of his newest salesman. He then wrote out a check for $50, which he explained was an advance on his first month's salary, and also handed him an envelope that contained a round-trip train ticket to Muskogee, Indian Territory.

It was his first train ride, and Bruce's heart beat a little faster as he stood on the platform of the Fayetteville station, heard the shrill whistle, and saw a column of smoke down the track. Soon the massive engine was pulling up in front of the excited passengers, belching out black smoke from its tall stack and hissing white steam from beneath its belly. It was a thrilling sight to behold, and Bruce marveled at how the wonders of modern engineering were changing the world in which he lived.

As he sat in the plush purple velvet seat, looking out the window as the landscape sped by, Bruce could not help but feel a sense of satisfaction. In the nine years since his father's death, he had been able to help support his mother and sister so that they were able to keep their farm until his mother remarried. He had earned degrees in education and business, had tried his hand at teaching in two schools, and was now entering the business world as a salesman. His mother seemed to be happy in her new life and now had two infant daughters—his half-sisters—named Ona and Ollie. Floy had met a young man by the name of Napoleon Bratton to whom she was betrothed. His grandfather Leslie was still living in the town that bore his name, and his surviving aunts and uncles were healthy and prosperous. Life was good. Bruce felt a profound sense of gratitude toward the Source of his blessings, and he closed his eyes and said a prayer of thanks.

The first thing he discovered about Muskogee, even before his train pulled into the station, was the origin of the town's name. He had struck up a conversation with a fellow traveling salesman who was returning to Indian Territory to sell farm equipment to the rapidly expanding population of settlers. His companion seemed rather knowledgeable about their destination, so Bruce asked him if he happened to know how the town got its name.

"Well sir, that's a right interesting matter," the salesman said. "Seems like Muskogee is another name for Creek. You'll hear some folks referring to the Indians in these parts as the Creek Nation and others calling 'em the Muskogee Nation. Don't seem to make no difference which you use; they mean the same thing. Anyway, I reckon that's how the town got its name."

Bruce was thanking his fellow traveler for the information, when the train's whistle blew and the passengers looked out their windows to see Muskogee station coming into view. There was an air of excitement as the weary travelers stepped down onto the station platform to be greeted by friends and relatives or to move on with their business. With his cloth knapsack slung over his back, Bruce said goodbye to his traveling companion and headed into the town. He had learned that Muskogee was one of the main centers of activity for the Creek Nation, and he could see that it was undergoing a transition from simple wooden stores to multiple-level red brick and stone buildings. Like most frontier towns, though, the streets were still dirt. They were now dusty, but he knew they would become quagmires when it rained. Wooden sidewalks lined the fronts of most of the stores and buildings, providing some protection for shoes and for ladies' long skirts from the perils of the dust and mud. And typical of most towns of the day were the hitching posts up and down the town's main street, many with horses patiently waiting with their wagons and buggies.

One of the buildings that seemed to be of the older generation was a two-story, white frame structure with a weathered sign over the door that identified it as the GENERAL STORE. Bruce headed toward it to pick up some supplies before renting a horse at the livery and then venturing out into the countryside to begin selling his fruit trees. Entering the store, he noticed that the clerk behind the counter was a young man about his own age. His black hair, light brown complexion, and facial features suggested that he was a member of the Creek Nation, like many of the people he had seen since his arrival. When the clerk looked up to see his newest customer, he gave Bruce a friendly smile.

"Just get in town?" the young man asked.

"Yes," Bruce replied. "Came in on the Katy train from Fayetteville. Bruce Leslie's the name," he said, extending his hand.

"Jake McIntosh," the young man replied, taking his hand and giving it a firm shake. "What brings you to Muskogee?"

"Well, sir, I represent Bently & Cobb Nursery, and we're introducing a new line of fruit trees to the area."

Jake nodded and thought for a moment. "Ought to do well 'round here," he said with a sincere expression. "Lots of new settlers comin' in, and I reckon they'll be wantin' to have fruit trees on their farms."

Bruce smiled and was very grateful for the encouraging word and for a friendly face. From Jake's last name, Bruce assumed that he was one of the half-bloods he had heard about. So, after a moment of silence, he took a chance on a bit of levity.

"My folks originally came from Scotland, and from your name I reckon some of yours did too, so maybe we're somehow connected," he said with a chuckle.

Jake gave a friendly laugh and appeared to take no offense. "Well, you may be right. I do have Scottish ancestry. When the Scots came to Georgia, they married into my Creek family. I'm what they call mixed-blood, like most of the Creeks 'round here. There are still a lot of full-blood Creeks about, but most of 'em live to the west of us."

The two young men again allowed moments of silence to pass, as they both sensed a feeling of friendship developing.

"So what are your plans from here?" Jake finally ventured.

"Well, I need to buy some supplies from you and then go to the livery to rent a horse. Then I reckon I'll head out into the countryside to begin visiting the farms and showing them our line of trees."

"Got a place to stay?" Jake asked.

Bruce shook his head. His plans hadn't gotten that far yet, but the folks back at Bently & Cobb had suggested he might sleep in whatever barns or huts the farmers could provide.

"Why don't you come to our house tonight?" Jake offered. "You can have dinner with us and tell my Dad about your trees. I suspect he'd like to have some fruit trees on our farm. We have a place out back where you can stay and then get a proper start in the morning."

Bruce couldn't believe his good fortune. He sincerely thanked Jake and told him that he would be most grateful to accept his kind offer. As he walked out of the general store, he paused for a second on the wooden sidewalk and again offered a silent prayer of thanks.

Riding out toward the McIntosh farm in the late afternoon, Bruce wondered what he would find there. Growing up, he had heard stories of the American Indians that did not suggest initiative or prosperity. But he was soon surprised to find himself riding up a long private road lined by large shade trees toward a stately farmhouse. Jake met him at the front door and brought him in to a well-appointed living room where he introduced him to his parents and younger siblings. Bruce's preconceived notions of the inhabitants of Indian Territory was suddenly challenged as he was greeted by the courteous and cultured occupants of the home.

The dinner that evening was delicious, reminding Bruce how hungry he was and how much he had missed home cooking. During the conversation over dinner, he learned that most of their vast acreage on the McIntosh farm had been given to the family by the federal government when Jake's great-grandfather voluntarily led Creeks from Georgia in the early part of the century. Over the years, the family had acquired additional land and also had several businesses in town, including the general store.

After dinner, the men went into the parlor, where Jake's father studied the Bently & Cobb catalogue of fruit trees and placed Bruce's first order, much to his delight. Mr. McIntosh then continued explaining the history of his people with an obvious concern for the changes that were occurring.

"My great-grandfather, Chief William McIntosh, was the principal chief of the Lower Creeks in Georgia back during the first part of the century. Being a half-blood of Native and Scottish heritage, he was able to work with both sides, and he believed that the best hope for the Indians was to cooperate with the white settlers. But the Upper Creek full-bloods would have no part of it. One night, a band of them dragged the Chief from his home, killed him on his front lawn, and burned down his home. His son, Chilly McIntosh, assumed the leadership and began voluntary migration of Lower Creeks into the Indian Territory that was provided for in the government's 1830 Act.

"For nearly a half-century," Mr. McIntosh continued, "the Creek Nation and the other four nations, or what the whites like to call the 'civilized tribes,' were allowed to function as autonomous nations here in Indian Territory. Then, about ten years ago, things started to change. White settlers began occupying land that was not specifically allocated to the tribes. Some people called them Boomers. At first, the federal troops ran them off, but more just kept coming and finally they were declared to be legal and allowed to stake claims on land that the federal government opened as 'unassigned land.' That was the beginning of what they like to call the 'great land rush.' The first was about four years ago, in 1889, and there have been several more since. Just a few months ago, they had one of the biggest up north in Cherokee country. Now they're starting to talk about turning our land into a state of the United States. Already the northwestern half of Indian Territory, created by the land runs, is being referred to as Oklahoma Territory. And then what will become of our people?"

It was obviously a rhetorical question, and the men sat for a while in grim silence. Bruce felt especially uncomfortable, as he began to understand what his people were perpetrating on Jake's people. Mr. McIntosh apparently recognized the embarrassing situation in which he had put his guest and broke the tension with a casual laugh and an answer to his own question.

"Our ancestors have prospered because they did not attempt to fight the white man, as did some of our brothers, but sought to live in peace and adjust to the changes that are beyond our power to influence. And that is the way we must continue to exist. And hopefully, with God's guidance, we will find a way that all people can live together in peace and prosperity."

Bruce awoke as the first pale light of dawn filtered through the guesthouse window. He found that the McIntosh family was already up, tending to their chores and preparing for another busy day. Over a hearty breakfast, Jake and his father gave him some suggestions of other farms in the area that might be good customers for his fruit trees and provided him with the directions. Bruce asked if he could give them a hand with the farm work before he headed out, but they insisted that he should be about his own work. And so he saddled his horse, thanked his generous hosts as sincerely as he knew how and headed off down the road, having no idea how their paths would cross again in the years to come.

He soon realized that his good fortune had peaked rather early in his career as a traveling salesman. Most of the farmers he met in the Muskogee area were courteous, or at least civil, although none gave him the special attention that he had received from the McIntosh family. It soon became clear to him that he had not only stumbled fortuitously into one of the most generous families in the Creek Nation, but also one of the most respected, at least among the half-bloods of the tribe. The few full-bloods he met had less to say about the McIntoshes, and some even made disparaging comments. And the white settlers that he met in the area didn't even seem to know much about them—or care.

The farms also varied considerably; those of the half-blood Creeks appeared the more prosperous, although none quite comparing with the McIntosh farm. Bruce's sleeping arrangements also went downhill after that first night. Some farms had huts where he was allowed to spend the night and others put him up in their barns, although there were other nights that he slept under the stars. He also discovered that reaching some of the farms meant fording the Arkansas River, for which he was glad to have a steady and reliable horse. But, on the whole, he was pleased with his success during the first weeks on the job. He had been able to place several more orders for his fruit trees, which he mailed to Bently & Cobb from the Muskogee post office. Then he turned west to head deeper into Indian Territory.

As he rode along in solitude, Bruce began to notice a change in both the landscape of the country and its inhabitants. The terrain was becoming a bit more rolling and wooded, which reminded him somewhat of his home back in Leslie and gave him a sense of comfort.

But there was also a feeling of loneliness about the land. He would ride for long stretches with no signs of civilization, and the farms he did encounter were quite isolated and extremely modest. He stopped at every one of them in the hope of making a sale, although his success seemed to progressively diminish the farther west he went. Most of the farmers appeared to be full-blood Indians or white settlers who had recently arrived, and neither group was particularly welcoming of a new face around their property. Bruce also came to realize that most of the people in this area were quite poor and unable to purchase fruit trees even if they had wanted to. Nevertheless, he was able to make a few sales and found that his friendly nature was usually reciprocated and that even those who had no money to buy his trees were willing to provide him a place to sleep in a barn or hut, and some even shared their meager meals with him.

Looking back on it, Bruce would remember those days as some of the loneliest in his life. And yet he felt a strange sense of peace to be all alone in this new country, which he increasingly found to be beautiful. Sometimes he would pull his horse off to the side of the dirt road, dismount, and sit for awhile, looking out across the countryside and wondering what it might be like someday as people continued to fill it up. Aside from his fruit tree catalogue, the only other book he carried in his knapsack was his Bible—the one his father had given him. In those moments of quiet solitude, he would often get it out and read a few passages. As he read, he would become aware of the wind rustling the leaves in the tress above him and swirling around his head. And it always reminded him that he was never alone.

About thirty-five miles west of Muskogee, Bruce realized that he was approaching the outskirts of another town. The farms were becoming more numerous and closer together, and most were decidedly more prosperous than those he had just visited. At one of the farms, he encountered a man with dark skin and a dignified, reserved demeanor, who Bruce assumed was a full-blood Creek. When he explained the purpose of his visit, the man seemed to warm up a bit and even offered him a drink of cold water from his well. The two men sat together for a while, as the farmer flipped through the

Bently & Cobb catalogue. Bruce finally felt comfortable enough to ask about the community he was entering.

"When our fathers first come to this land, they hold grand council with other tribes beside flowing water west of here, called Deep Fork. In time, land beside flowing water become new capital of Creek Nation. Water remind fathers of river in ancestral land far to the east, called Creek word for 'bubbling water' – Okmulgee."

Bruce had never heard the name before but was just glad to be back in civilization where he could replenish his supplies and hopefully sell more of his fruit trees. After thanking the farmer for his hospitality and his order for a dozen apple trees, he headed on down the road toward the town of Okmulgee. As he passed other farms, he noted their locations, but decided to stop at them on another day, since he was anxious to reach the town before dark.

As he approached the center of the community, he was surprised to find that it was built around a large common green on which sat an impressive stone building. It was a square two-story structure with a roof that sloped upward to the center on all sides and supported a louvered cupola topped off with a brass weathervane and eagle. Large oak doors on the front and back of the building were flanked by four tall windows on either side. Smaller doors opened onto railed balconies above the entrances and were flanked by eight more tall windows. A four-foot stone wall surrounded the building and grounds of the town square. Bruce recalled the farmer saying that Okmulgee was the capital of the Creek Nation and suspected that this building had something to do with that. At the moment, however, he was more concerned about restocking his supplies and was able to find a general store across the street from the town square.

Upon entering the store, he saw that the clerk behind the counter was an elderly gentleman with long, gray, braided hair, and an appearance that suggested he was probably a full-blood Creek. Recalling his good fortune at the general store in Muskogee, Bruce walked up to the man, extended his hand and cheerfully introduced himself. But there was no response. The man seemed to recognize his presence, but neither looked at him nor said a word. After an awkward moment of silence, Bruce took a different tack and told the clerk, in a business-like manner, what he wished to purchase. The man grunted, turned his back to his customer and appeared to feel his way along the shelves of merchandise. It was then that Bruce realized the man must be blind and never saw his attempt at congeniality. Under the circumstances, he was surprised when the clerk returned with all the correct items and rang up the bill. Bruce handed him the money and, as the man carefully felt and counted each coin, he spoke for the first time.

"You new in town?"

"Yes sir," he replied. "I'm from Arkansas and been selling fruit trees in the region for the past month or so."

The clerk nodded but didn't appear impressed and seemed to have nothing more to say. Bruce assumed their conversation was over and was about to take his bag and leave, when he couldn't resist venturing one final comment.

"That's a mighty impressive building across the street."

The comment seemed to strike a chord with the clerk, as his sightless eyes appeared to light up with sense of pride. He nodded again, although this time with a bit more enthusiasm, and after a long silence, during which he seemed to be remembering something from the distant past, he cleared his throat and began to speak.

"Many moons ago, after war of states, our fathers come to Deep Fork for council of tribes. Make new laws to heal divide between our people. Build Council House of logs. Call new capital Okmulgee. Council have two bodies. I serve in House of Warriors. Other called House of Kings. Council House burn down. Replace with larger stone building."

Bruce looked out the window at the impressive structure and then back at the clerk, hoping to learn more. But that seemed to be the end of his lesson. The old man had turned away as though he had work to do. Bruce thanked him and walked out onto the wooden sidewalk. As he stood there for a moment, looking at the Creek Council House, he could not in his wildest dreams imagine that one day his picture would have a place of honor in that imposing building.

With the day nearly spent, Bruce found a boarding house that rented rooms by the night and decided to splurge with his dwindling bankroll, as he desperately wanted a good night of sleep and—

even more importantly—a place to wash up. Later that evening, he walked around the town and happened to pass the Methodist Church a couple of blocks off the town square. As the following day was Sunday, he decided to attend their service. And so, on a bright Sunday morning, feeling refreshed and clean for the first time in nearly a month, he stepped into the sanctuary just before 11 a.m. and seated himself in a back-row pew. Of course, he didn't know a soul in the congregation, but somehow he felt more at home than he had since leaving Arkansas, especially when he joined in singing the old familiar hymns. The preacher was not much older than Bruce but delivered a spirited sermon and was very friendly when the two shook hands at the end of the service.

For the next six days, he visited all the farms he could around Okmulgee. He found that the majority of the population were Creeks, both full-blood and mixed-blood, although there were also a growing number of white settlers. As he rode between farms, he found himself being drawn more and more to the rolling, wooded landscape, which continued to remind him so much of his home. And, when he came to the Deep Fork River, the swiftly flowing water brought back memories of his childhood when he, Eb, and Floy swam and fished in the streams of the Ozarks.

When he returned to the Methodist Church the following Sunday, he felt even more at home, in part because several members of the congregation were among the farmers he had met as he had traveled around selling his trees. He was impressed that the preacher remembered his name, and he enjoyed chatting with him and with the farmers he had come to know. They were all quite friendly and spoke highly of their growing community, as though they were hoping Bruce might stay. He explained that he would soon be returning to Arkansas, but that he would be around for one more Sunday service.

The following Sunday, he took his usual seat in the back row and nodded to a few of his new acquaintances. When the young preacher began his sermon, Bruce was interested to hear him begin with a passage from the book of Philippians: "...*this one thing I do, forgetting those things which are behind, and reaching forth unto those things which are before.*" When Bruce had talked with the preacher the previous Sunday, he had mentioned that he didn't know what he would be doing with his life, and he couldn't help but wonder if the sermon was directed at him. In any case, he listened intently as the preacher spoke of making the most of our God-given talents and how each one of us has the opportunity to make a difference in this world. Bruce thought he saw a twinkle in the preacher's eyes as they shook hands for the last time, and he somehow knew that the message he had just heard would challenge him for the rest of his life.

He thought about that last sermon many times as he rode back to Muskogee. During pauses along the way to rest both horse and rider, he would take out his Bible and reread the passages that the preacher had used. He knew that God had blessed him with certain talents, and he knew that he wanted to do something worthwhile with his life, but he simply could not see far enough ahead to know what that might be. On many occasions during the return trip, whether resting by the roadside or sitting on his horse, Bruce prayed that God would reveal to him the course that his life should take.

When he reached Muskogee, he went to the post office to mail his latest orders back to Bently & Cobb and was surprised to find a letter waiting for him that had been forwarded from his employers. It was from two of his cousins and was postmarked Denver, Colorado:

> Dear Bruce,
>
> This is a great town. Many opportunities. You would love it. Why not come visit us and see for yourself. You can stay with us a long as you wish.
>
> Your Cousins,
>
> Elmer and Lester

All the way home on the train, Bruce kept thinking about the sermon and his musings about his future and now the letter, which spoke of "opportunities." Was this God's response to his prayers? How else would he ever know without giving it a try? By the time his train pulled into Fayetteville station, he had made up his mind. He would use some of the money he had earned from his brief career as a fruit tree salesman to buy a train ticket to Denver, Colorado.

CHAPTER 6

Denver
1894–1902

BRUCE LESLIE HAD NEVER EXPERIENCED anything like it. He truly feared for his life. The spiders were as big as a man's hand. Bigger. They slithered like menacing shadows up the walls and across the ceiling, appearing ready to attack at any moment. And he could hear the giant rats, with their sharp teeth, gnawing on the wood in the attic above him, trying to break into his room. Outside, he could make out the sinister voices of those who wished him harm. They seemed to be laughing at the misery being inflicted on him, and he feared they would come bursting through the door any second.

He seemed unable to do anything about it. His body felt paralyzed as he lay in a pool of perspiration with every muscle aching and trembling and his vision fading in and out. "Is this why I was brought to Denver?" he wondered. Had he misread God's intention for him? Surely this was not the divine plan for how his life was to end. He tried to pray, but his fear and pain were so overwhelming that he seemed incapable of concentrating on anything else. "How could it have come to this," he agonized, "when it had all started out so well?"

The clicking and clacking of metal wheels on the steel rails intensified as the door of the passenger car swung open and the conductor stepped in. He gripped the back of a seat to steady himself against the swaying of the train and, when the door was again closed, announced in a loud voice, "Folks, we have just passed over the state line into Colorado and should be pullin' into Denver station in about four more hours."

Bruce looked out the window, hoping to see the Rocky Mountains on the horizon, but the landscape was still flat and featureless for as far as he could see. It had been like this for much of the fifteen hours that he had been traveling. After leaving Fayetteville station in Arkansas the day before, his train had headed due north through Missouri until it entered the massive Kansas City station. This was his first exposure to a truly large city, and he found the size of the station both intimidating and exciting. But he had little time to consider his emotions as he stood, stretched his stiff legs, slung his satchel over his shoulder, and followed the other passengers, who were looking for their connections. His was on the Kansas Pacific line that would be heading due west through the entire state of Kansas into Colorado to the Denver station.

Having lived most of his twenty years in the green, rolling hills of the Ozarks, he had no idea that any place could be so flat and barren. Hour upon hour, as they rode through Kansas, he saw nothing but the flattest farmland without a single tree. The farms he saw, however, appeared to be reasonably prosperous, and the land was clearly fertile, with cultivated fields that stretched farther than any he could have ever imagined. But the wide openness of the land and its stark difference from all that he had known before gave him a sense of loneliness, and he wondered if he was already becoming homesick.

A couple of hours after the conductor's announcement that they had crossed into Colorado, Bruce thought he saw something on the far horizon. It was hard to tell, at first, if his eyes were playing tricks on him. He was not sure whether he was seeing distant clouds or actual land masses erupting from the flat landscape. But, as the train continued rumbling down the tracks, the masses began to change from faint gray hues to deepening blues and to assume more definite forms. It eventually became clear that he was indeed looking at the majestic Rocky Mountains. And the landscape outside his window was turning greener, with increasingly dense woodlands. The trees differed significantly from the stubby, sturdy oaks back in the Ozarks. These had tall, straight trunks with a light gray bark that appeared almost white in the sunlight and rich green leaves that fluttered in the gentle afternoon breeze.

As the train pulled into the impressive Denver station, with its many parallel tracks and trains coming and going from all parts of the country, Bruce again marveled at the wonder of this modern age of transportation. But he also took a moment to close his eyes and say a prayer of thanks for a safe and pleasant journey. When he opened his eyes, he saw all the people standing on the platform to greet the arrivals, and his heart soared when he saw among them his two cousins, Elmer and Lester, grinning and waving at him.

During his first few days in Denver, Bruce rented a horse and buggy to explore the city and the foothills of the Rockies to the west. His cousins, with whom he was staying, joined him when they could, but he was on his own most of the time and enjoyed studying the natural beauty of the area and the architecture and history of the city. He learned that Denver began with the gold rush of 1859, when fortune seekers converged on an area near the junction of Cherry Creek and the South Platte River. However, the gold yield was not plentiful in those early years, and the nascent settlement was plagued by fires, floods, Indian wars, and the discovery of gold elsewhere. Nevertheless, it survived and was designated the capital of the territory in 1867, a distinction it retained after statehood in 1876. When the Transcontinental Railroad linked the country from east to west in the '70s, it bypassed the still relatively small community of Denver, but the citizens of the town raised enough money to build a line that connected them with the transcontinental line at Cheyenne. This proved to be an economic boon for the city, which grew from fewer than 5,000 citizens to a population, by the time Bruce arrived, of more than 100,000.

For a young man from Arkansas. it was a vibrant, exciting, and terribly large town—in fact, Bruce found the size a bit intimidating and couldn't help but wonder how he would fare in such a place. But it was not so much his first impressions of the big city that captivated him as it was the natural beauty that lay to the west of town. As the land rose up into the foothills of the Rocky Mountains, the trees he had seen from the train became increasingly abundant. He learned that they were called aspen, and he could see that some at higher elevations were already showing the yellow color of their leaves, with which the entire landscape would be awash come fall. But what struck him with the greatest sense of awe were the stark, jagged mountains that rose high above the timberline. The enormous, barren peaks were in striking contrast to the low, green, gently rolling hills of the Ozarks, which reminded him of how far he was from home.

Cousin Elmer worked for the leading newspaper in the city, the *Denver Post*, and told Bruce of a position that had just opened up there in the circulation department. It wasn't entirely clear to him what "circulation" encompassed, but Bruce could see himself sitting behind a desk, typing out the stories of the day, or going out on assignment and hurrying back with the latest scoop. In any case, with the bankroll from his days as a traveling salesman running low, he needed to get back to the ranks of the employed, and this sounded like an excellent opportunity. His interview in the employment department seemed to go well, and, much to his delight, he was offered the job. It was then that reality set in as he learned the specifics of his new position, which was to deliver the papers—in other words, he would be a paperboy.

After the initial letdown, Bruce decided it wasn't all that bad. Sure, he would have to get up well before the crack of dawn to deliver the morning edition, but he was quite accustomed to rising early, and it would give him time during the day for other pursuits before returning to deliver the evening papers. Another benefit was the issuance of a company bicycle, which would give him a much-needed means of transportation, although he soon learned that his salary was "adjusted" to compensate for this expense. The position also introduced him to his first circle of friends, the other paperboys, and he became a member of the "Denver Carrier Club." A few of these young men, like himself, were motivated by higher ambitions and were willing to do whatever it took to achieve their goals in life. Some had already matriculated into programs of higher education and were working to put themselves through school. Others seemed to have already reached the summit of their ambition. They were a bit rougher and tougher-talking and swore to never again darken the door of a school. But Bruce found that he liked them all and soon became friendly with each of his fellow carriers.

The first few weeks were actually quite pleasant, as the sun rose early, and he enjoyed being out in the warmth of the morning. He would ride his bike to the newspaper office and sit with the other young men, folding the papers and putting them in cloth bags that hung over the handlebars. Then he would head off on his morning delivery route. He was usually finished by midmorning and would go back to the boardinghouse that he was sharing with his cousins, for a bite of breakfast. This gave him several hours to read, write letters to the folks back home, or explore the city and the countryside, before returning to the *Post* to repeat the procedure on his evening route. He would get back just in time to join the others around the boardinghouse table for a hearty supper. It didn't take long for him to adjust to this routine and he soon found himself rather enjoying it—until the weather changed.

It seemed to Bruce as though the change occurred overnight. One morning, he woke up to find that it was dark and cold outside. Getting out of a warm bed was now more of a challenge, although he found the cold air to be invigorating once he was out and moving about. Temperatures often got quite low in the Ozarks when he was growing up, and he told himself that he could handle the Denver weather. But the days kept getting colder, and then the snows began. His jacket seemed totally inadequate, and he layered on every piece of clothing he had, but still the icy chill penetrated into his bones. He hated to waste his money, but finally succumbed to spending a dollar on a heavy coat at a used clothing store. And so he struggled through his first months of a Denver winter.

Long before deciding on his move to Denver, the question that was foremost on his mind was what to do with the rest of his life. Whatever direction that might be, he knew he needed to strengthen his liberal studies. So he took the opportunity to sign up for some courses at Dix Normal School. Most of his classes were in the late morning or early afternoon between his two delivery times, although he had occasional classes at night. He enjoyed courses in English and mathematics as well as history and geography, but the subject that appealed to him most was science. He looked forward to all his classes, not only for the chance to come in out of the cold and sit in a warm, well-lit room, but especially for the opportunity to stimulate his mental faculties after the mind-numbing hours of delivering newspapers. And yet, even as he expanded the horizons of his knowledge, he still could not see far enough into the future to know what he would one day do with his education.

That first Christmas away from home was hard for all three cousins. None of them could afford the money or the time away from their jobs to make the trip back to Arkansas, but they were thankful to have each other to be with during the holy season. Bruce had not been in Denver long before he discovered the church where he felt most comfortable. It was not a Presbyterian or Methodist church of his heritage, but a mission church, called the People's Tabernacle Congregational Church, under the leadership of Reverend Thomas Uzzell. Before long, Bruce would take an active role in the life of the church, but on his first Christmas Eve away from home, he sat in the back of the sanctuary listening to the old familiar Bible stories, singing along to the traditional Christmas carols, and thinking about his mother and siblings and all the dear souls back in Arkansas.

That first Denver winter finally passed, and Bruce felt the reinvigoration in his heart that invariably comes with the harbingers of spring—the crocus and daffodils breaking through the last icy layers of snow, the tender young leaves budding out on the aspens and beginning to flutter in the gentle spring breeze, and the wonderful warmth of the sun breaking through the final gray of winter's clouds. There had been times, on those dark mornings with the snow biting his face, when he had considered giving up and returning home. Even the classrooms had become tedious, possibly because he was so deprived of sleep. His two delivery routes each day took longer in the winter, leaving him just enough time for his classes. And then he had to stay up late every night with the requisite homework, only to rise before the first sign of morning light to start the whole routine again. But his hard work paid dividends, and he completed all his courses with honors. With a couple more hours of summer school, he would have the equivalent of an undergraduate degree. And yet he continued to wonder where all this was taking him.

Bruce had struggled for many years with the question of God's purpose for his life. As he grew older, he became increasingly concerned about his indecision, and he prayed each day for discernment. He thought about the ministry and discussed it with Rev. Uzzell, but somehow he just couldn't convince himself that this was his primary calling. He remembered how the study of science had interested him but wasn't sure how to channel that into his vocation. His thoughts frequently went back to those days in Indian Territory, and he recalled the pleasure that he derived as a salesman, possibly because he enjoyed being around people. Maybe he was meant to be a businessman. In any case, when the next fall arrived, Bruce enrolled in courses at DeSoller's Business School as he continued to work for the *Denver Post*.

The months seemed to fly by faster and faster as he tried to balance his work and his studies. He saved every penny he could and was finally able to afford a room of his own and to send a little money home to his mother. About the only diversions from his work and study that he allowed himself were attending church and writing letters to his mother and other relatives. He especially enjoyed receiving news from home, most of which was good, although in 1896 he was notified of the death of his grandfather, Samuel Leslie, who had lived eighty-seven years, thirty as a widower. The three cousins desperately wanted to be home to mourn with their kin, but they consoled each other by recalling their grandfather's remarkable life as the leading citizen of the town that now bore his name. As Bruce thought about a life that was so fulfilling, he was reminded once again of how blessed he was to have such a distinguished heritage, but it also rekindled the nagging question of where his own life was headed and how his progeny would one day remember him.

Although Bruce had no way of knowing it, the answer to his question was not far off. But it would come in a way that he could never have imagined. After completing his studies at the business school, he decided it was time to leave the *Post* and take a more promising job with the Denver mercantile company of Daniels & Fisher. For the rest of his days, Bruce would look back on that decision as the worst in his life—and the best.

He had not been at Daniels & Fisher long before one of his fellow workers, with whom he was in close contact each day, developed what appeared to be an especially bad cold. His coughing was becoming increasingly severe, and he was complaining of chills and headaches. Sick leave was frowned upon, and the young man was reluctant to stay home for fear of losing his job. But, on the fifth day of his symptoms, just as Bruce had begun to notice red spots on his colleague's forehead and cheeks, the fellow did not show up for work. No one thought too much about it, and everyone went on with their daily tasks. About a week later, however, Bruce began to feel a bit feverish. That night, as he lay in the bed of his small boardinghouse room, he felt a severe chill from which no amount of blankets provided relief. By the following morning, he had developed a cough and was starting to feel a soreness in his mouth. Like his fellow worker, he did not feel that he could afford to stay home, so he pushed on. After another three days, however, he began to notice the same red spots on his face that he had seen on his colleague. He decided it was time to visit the company doctor, who instantly recognized that Bruce had measles. The doctor gave him a bottle of medicine to ease his cough and the soreness in his mouth and told him that he must go home immediately and stay there for at least a week so as not to transmit the highly contagious disease to any of his fellow workers. He would arrange for a local doctor to call on him that evening and to follow him until he recovered.

Bruce did as he was instructed, but before going to his room, he stopped by his landlady's apartment and slid a note under her door, telling of his situation. He then went upstairs and gladly crawled into bed, praying that his symptoms would soon pass. Before long, there was a knock on his door, and he was surprised to see his landlady come in as though she had no fear of contracting the disease. She explained that she had had the measles as a child and now seemed to be immune to it. She was a kind lady and told Bruce that she would check on him from time to time and bring his meals up to his room, for which he expressed immense gratitude. He must have slept a bit after that, for it had grown darker outside his window when he heard another knock at the door. Before he could respond, the door opened and a tall, portly man wearing a dark, three-piece suit and a silk tie walked in. His hair was gray and thinning and bags of skin hung beneath his eyes, which looked weary but also conveyed a sense of compassion. He did not smile, and yet there was a distinct impression of warmth in his dignified, business-like manner. He took the few short steps from the door to where Bruce lay, placed his black bag on a chair beside the bed, and introduced himself as Dr. Burr.

By now, Bruce was feeling truly rotten. The spots on his face and neck had grown darker and had spread to other parts of his body. His breathing was labored, he had a splitting headache, and the inside of his mouth felt raw and sore. Through red, swollen eyes, he looked up at the blurry silhouette of the imposing figure above him, which struck him as having an almost saintly quality—this man of great learning and compassion, who had the power to heal him of his terrible affliction. And the gentle, reassuring tone of the doctor's voice gave him an added sense of comfort.

"Feeling pretty bad are you, son?" he asked. Bruce could only nod. "Well, let's take a look."

Dr. Burr took his patient's temperature and checked his pulse. He looked inside his mouth and noted the telltale eruptions. Then he carefully examined the spots on his face and chest. He pressed on one, which caused it to momentarily blanch, but quickly fill back up with blood. This latter sign seemed especially troubling to the doctor, who frowned and paused as if to contemplate its significance.

"Is it measles, doctor?" Bruce was finally able to ask with a raspy voice.

The doctor nodded, as he reached into his bag for a bottle of medicine. "And I'm afraid it's the rough kind, son. There are different types of measles. The mild form comes and goes in about three days. But yours is a bit more serious. In fact, you have a type called black measles, because the spots on your skin turn dark with blood."

Bruce probably heard less than half of what the doctor was telling him. His only concern was getting better. Dr. Burr told him that the medicine he was prescribing would help with his fever and pain and told him how often to take it. He said it would also be important for Bruce to follow a strict diet, which he would discuss with the landlady. He promised to return the following day and then rose and took his leave.

No one could ever say with certainty whether it was the severity of his condition or an unusual reaction to the medication, but that night Bruce slipped into a state of altered consciousness. It was not a peaceful sleep that freed him from his agony, but a convulsive feeling of things going from bad to worse. Now, in addition to his physical misery, his life seemed in peril from giant spiders and rats that infested his room and merciless intruders who lurked just outside his door. He struggled in vain to rise from his bed so that he could defend himself, but something seemed to be holding him back. The harder he tried the more hopeless his situation seemed to become. The voices outside the room were growing louder, and now the door was opening and they were coming for him. He tried to scream, but no sound came from his mouth. And now they were calling his name.

"Bruce, Bruce!" A hand reached out from the voice and grabbed his arm. He tried to free himself but realized that he had no strength. "Bruce, Bruce," the voice came again. "It's all right." There was something familiar about the voice. Through slits in his swollen lids, light entered his feverish eyes with the outline of a face silhouetted against the light. He struggled to focus on the face, which faded in and out of view but gradually became clearer until he finally realized that he was looking up into the worried face of his cousin Elmer. He was still confused and unable to talk and feared for the safety of his cousin in this dangerous room. But, when he looked around him, there were no spiders on the walls, and the sounds of the rats had vanished. He seemed to be alone in the room except for Elmer and, standing quietly in the doorway, Dr. Burr. As the cobwebs in his mind began to clear, Bruce felt his body slowly relaxing.

Elmer told him that he had been unresponsive for nearly three days, and they had all feared for his life. His landlady had been a saint, he said, coming in frequently to check on him. The doctor had told them that it was one of the worst cases of black measles he had seen, but he seemed to be more optimistic that morning, noting that Bruce's temperature was returning to normal and his lungs were clearing. Since he was no longer contagious, Elmer stayed with his cousin for the rest of the day, and they were joined that afternoon by Lester.

Dr. Burr returned in the evening and happily confirmed that indeed his patient seemed to be on the road to recovery.

"You gave us quite a fright, son," he told his patient. "For a while there, I truthfully wasn't sure if you were going to make it. But you seem to have a strong constitution. It looks like God must have plans for your life."

Those last words were spoken with a twinkle in the doctor's eyes, and for the first time in many days Bruce was able to manage a weak smile. After his cousins and Dr. Burr were gone, the landlady came up with a cup of broth, which tasted delicious after such a long fast. Then he was alone again and lay in his bed, contemplating the tumultuous events that had just rocked his life. Most of all, he thought about the doctor's final words. Bruce had no doubt that God had plans for his life, and yet he still had the frustrating sense of looking into a crystal ball and seeing only mist. But something had shaken him during his recent trial, as though a gentle wind were beginning to blow away the mist and would soon bring his future into focus.

The following day, Dr. Burr returned to check on his patient and was again delighted to find that he was making steady improvement. After completing a brief examination, the elderly doctor settled himself in the straight wooden chair beside Bruce's bed and sat quietly and pensively for a few minutes before sharing what was on his mind.

"So, Bruce, what are you planning to do now with the rest of your life?"

"Well, sir, I don't rightly know," Bruce began, surprised to be asked the question that was foremost on his own mind. "I've been asking myself that very question now for a number of years. I've tried my hand at teaching and business and enjoyed them both, but something just seemed to be missing. I've thought about the ministry, but so far I haven't really felt the calling. I've surely prayed about it a lot but am still waiting for God to show me his plan."

The old doctor did not respond immediately but sat quietly as though he was respectfully considering all that his young patient had said. Then he fixed his eyes directly into Bruce's eyes and, with the faint suggestion of a smile, he said the words that would forever change the life of Bruce Leslie.

"Have you thought about medicine?"

"Me? A doctor?" Although his response sounded a bit incredulous, the truth is that it was not the first time the thought had crossed

Bruce's mind. He greatly admired his Uncle John, who had a successful medical practice back in Arkansas, and he had enjoyed his science courses as much as any subject in his formal training. And then there were the events of the last few days, which had taught him how profoundly a physician can enter into the intimate life of his patients and bring them healing and hope. But aspiring to a medical education had seemed to him as remote as the moon, not only because of the cost, but also because of the difficulty of being accepted into a medical school. So he had never allowed himself to seriously consider the possibility.

Dr. Burr's smile broadened a bit, as though the response did not surprise him. "I've been checking up on you these last few days. Tom Uzzell at the Tabernacle is an old friend and speaks very highly of you. I also have friends at the *Post*, who have told me of your work ethic and collegiality. We need men like you in the medical profession."

Bruce did not know how to respond to such approbation, which always embarrassed him. He sat mute, with his eyes fixed on the good doctor, as though he anticipated that he had more to tell him—which he did.

"I'm on the faculty of the Denver Homeopathic Medical College."

"Homeo—what?" Bruce asked, having never heard the word.

Now the doctor burst into a hearty laugh. "Homeopathy is a relatively new philosophy of medicine that is becoming increasingly popular in America. In most ways it is like regular medical practice, except our treatments are gentler and more focused, and we are committed to both science and spirituality. The school here in Denver was just opened three years ago, and our first class graduated last year. If you're interested, I could arrange for you to meet with our admissions committee."

By now, Bruce's head was spinning. Had he heard correctly? Had he just been offered the chance to sit for a possible spot in a medical school? For a moment, the logistics of the proposition—such as how he could pay for it—seemed irrelevant, as he allowed the intoxicating thought of being "Dr. Leslie" to titillate his imagination. Looking back on it, he couldn't recall exactly what he had said to Dr. Burr, other than to thank him as sincerely as he knew how and to promise him that he would give his generous offer the most serious thought and prayer.

That night, as he lay in his bed, unable to sleep, he became increasingly excited as he considered this possible new direction in his life. Why had he not seen it before? The more he thought about it, the more convinced he became that this surely was what God had planned for him all along. Even his terrible illness, which almost killed him, must have been part of the plan, because it led him to Dr. Burr and to this pivotal moment in his life. As the first shaft of morning light filtered through his boardinghouse window, it was as though the wind had finally blown away the last of the mist in his crystal ball, and he could now see clearly where his life was heading.

Dr. Burr returned a couple of days later and was overjoyed when Bruce told him that he would be honored and grateful to appear before the medical school's admission committee. That meeting was arranged as soon as Bruce had regained sufficient strength. It went just as Dr. Burr suspected it would, and in the fall of 1898, Bruce Leslie matriculated to the Denver Homeopathic Medical College.

American medicine in the nineteenth century was gradually transitioning from the irrational practices of the eighteenth century—bloodletting, purging, blistering, leeches, and the like—toward a more rational approach based on clinical and laboratory science. Along the way, a number of alternative concepts were introduced for the health and healing of the human body. One of the most popular of these was homeopathy, the underlying principle of which was that "like cures like," or that medicines have curative powers which create symptoms similar to the disease being treated. It advocated using the lowest possible dose of a medication, prescribing only one drug at a time, and adhering to strict diets and exercise. Its appeal stemmed, in part, from the gentler, more patient-specific remedies, as compared to the harsh, often dangerous treatments of traditional medicine. Whatever the reasons, homeopathy acquired a particular appeal among middle- and upper-class American families, including such luminaries as Samuel F. B. Morse, Henry Wadsworth Longfellow, Harriet Beecher Stowe, Nathaniel Hawthorne, and President Chester A. Arthur. The American Institute of Homeopathy was founded in 1844, three years before the American Medical Association, and by the 1880s there were forty-four homeopathic medical schools in the United States. Bruce Leslie would always believe that Providence had brought him to the one in Denver.

In the months before he was scheduled to start medical school, Bruce did his best to arrange his life in a way that would be compatible with his educational demands, both in terms of money and time. There would be no financial support from home. In fact, shortly after the death of his grandfather, he received another letter informing him of the passing of his stepfather, David Marrs. This left his mother to support herself and her two young daughters on the meager income from the Marrs estate and whatever odd jobs she could find. Therefore, Bruce knew he would not only have to support himself entirely, but also send money home to his mother whenever he could.

He decided to return to his old job at the *Denver Post* because the early morning and late afternoon routes would allow him to attend all his classes during the day. In addition, it gave him the advantage of a company bicycle for the much-needed transportation. He also found new accommodations in the home of the county sheriff, Robert Jones, where he could pay for his room by working for the sheriff's wife. There was a rather tearful goodbye with his former landlady, who had been so kind to him, but she understood his need for frugality and wished him well. His loneliness in this new arrangement was soon lessened when Cousin Elmer also moved into the Jones home. They were joined in the house by two law students, and the four young men were given kitchen privileges and allowed to prepare their own meals, further reducing costs.

As the aspen trees began to turn their autumnal yellow and the chill of fall nipped the air, Bruce began the hardest four years of his life. Early each morning, he would fire up the furnace in the Jones house before leaving on his paper route, then sit in classes all day and get out just in time for his evening route. As soon as he got home, he would run errands and perform odd jobs for Mrs. Jones before preparing a quick dinner and then studying until late into the night. This was his daily routine for at least five days of every week, and the weekends were filled with more chores and intensive study. It seemed as if he could never keep up with all that he had to learn. And yet he found that he was loving it. Studying the anatomy and physiology of the human body in his first year of medical school filled him with a sense of awe at the wonder of creation and brought to mind one of his favorite passages from Psalms, "I will praise thee; for I am fearfully and wonderfully made."

His only reprieve from the study and work was attending People's Tabernacle Congregational Church every Sunday. By now, he was a well-known and active member of the church. They had a weekly newsletter, the *Tabernacle Good Samaritan*, a rather folksy four-page publication with detailed information about youth programs, Sunday School classes, health issues of the congregation, and the like. When the need arose for a new editor of the *Good Samaritan*, someone recalled that Bruce worked for the *Denver Post* and therefore probably knew something about journalism. In any case, he accepted the offer and served as editor for the remainder of his time in Denver, except for a brief absence that was explained in one issue of the newsletter: "Mr. Leslie, editor of our paper, has been seriously ill. We are glad to learn he has recovered and is able to be with us again."

A frequent feature of the *Good Samaritan* was poems, many of which came from the editor's collection of favorites. One of those was entitled "I Shall Not Pass This Way Again," which includes the verse: "If I this moment shall withhold / The help I might be giving, / Some soul may die, and I shall lose / The sweetest joy of living." This thought returned to Bruce many times, as he moved from the classroom to the clinical years of his medical training and began facing life-and-death issues. And it would stay with him throughout the half century that he did his best for all those who needed his healing touch.

As much as he had enjoyed the first two didactic years— normal anatomy and physiology in the first year and disease states in the second—it was the clinical years that made the practice of medicine come alive for Bruce. He learned to recognize and treat a dizzying number of infectious diseases, including cholera, typhoid, tuberculosis, smallpox, and—the one which had special significance to him—measles. He also learned how to set fractures, dress wounds, deliver babies, and many other procedures. Sometimes, in a single day, he would experience the exhilaration of witnessing a new life come into the world and also the heartache of seeing a soul depart when death triumphed over the medical knowledge of the day. These encounters, at the two extremes of human emotion, often left Bruce pondering the wonder and the mystery of the cycle of life.

In their final year, the senior medical students were assigned specific patients to care for, albeit under the watchful eye of their professor. One of these was a pretty little eight-year-old girl with auburn bangs and a serene smile. She had suffered the misfortune of having two rambunctious older brothers who decided to treat her to a ride down a steep hill in their homemade wagon. The vehicle came apart about halfway down the hill, and the child fell out and broke her leg. It was a severe fracture, and there was concern that she might never walk again. Bruce and two of his fourth-year classmates were assigned to her care. As gently as they could, they reset her bone and then applied a plaster cast. She remained in the hospital for many days as the anxious medical students hovered over her. When the cast finally came off, the bone was straight and strong. She would require crutches awhile longer, but eventually they could be discarded, and she would be as good as new. It was hard to say who was more elated, the patient and her family or the young doctors.

Throughout his four years of medical school, Bruce remained active in his church, not only editing the *Good Samaritan*, but also teaching a Sunday School class of teenage women. He had never lost his love for teaching, and he considered the privilege of sharing God's word to be the noblest of all educational endeavors. It was an opportunity that he would value and cherish for the remainder of his life. And he seemed to have an aptitude for it, at least according to an item in the weekly newsletter: "We notice increased attendance in Mr. Nichol's, Miss Mook's, and Mr. Leslie's classes. They are making their side of the house very populous." Part of Bruce's popularity may have come from the infatuation that his students had for their handsome medical student teacher. One person in particular who had an eye for Bruce was a young lady in her late teens by the name of Lula Mook. She had a sweet, oval face and curly blond hair that accented her blue eyes and cherry red lips. Her father was a wealthy businessman and one of the church's most generous benefactors. He saw to it that his beloved daughter was always dressed in the latest and finest fashions. Lula was cheerful and vivacious and did not lack for admirers among the young men. She taught a class of first- and second-graders and so was not able to attend Bruce's class. But, from time to time, she would get a friend to take charge of her class so she could attend his and hope that he noticed her.

Lula was not the only one who had her eye on Bruce Leslie. Her mother, Eva, was one of the pillars of the church. She was on just about every committee and could always be counted on to find time for one more task. In fact, she would make her disappointment known if she was not invited to be a part of whatever the church's latest endeavor might be. And no one wanted to disappoint Eva Mook, not only because of her husband's importance to the finances of the church, but also because of her influence over most of the decisions that were made by the congregation. But Eva's greatest concern was for the future of her daughter, who was approaching her eighteenth birthday and still had no serious matrimonial prospects. She shared Lula's impression of the handsome young medical student in their church and entertained fantasies of her daughter one day becoming "Mrs. Bruce Leslie, wife of Denver's most prosperous physician." There were other young women in the church who also dreamed of someday being so blessed, but Lula and Eva's aspirations had become common knowledge, which meant hands off for all the others. In fact, the only person who seemed totally oblivious to the whole matter was Bruce Leslie.

Despite his appreciation of the opposite sex, Bruce was extremely pragmatic and goal-oriented. He knew the day would come when he would want to find that special person with whom he could share his dreams and hopes and enjoy a warm and loving family. But first he had to complete his medical education and establish a successful practice. Until then, he had neither the time nor the money to think about courting. But his resolve would be challenged in the summer of 1900.

Eva received a letter in the spring of 1900 with news that thrilled Lula. It was from Eva's cousin, Nettie McKeage, whose family had recently moved from Hooper, Nebraska, to Leadville, Colorado. Ever since the move, the McKeages had been hoping to accept the Mooks' invitation to visit them in Denver. As the crow flies, Leadville is about eighty miles southwest of Denver, but the rail line wound through the Rockies along steep ridges carved into the high peaks and down into gorges between the mountains, making the trip nearly twice as long. So coming to Denver wasn't a simple weekend visit. But, since John McKeage worked for the railroad, he was able to obtain special fares for the family, and they had finally decided to make the trip that summer. The entire family could only stay for about a week, but what thrilled Lula was that their daughter, Blossom, would be allowed to accept the Mooks' invitation to spend the summer with them. Lula had never met her cousin, but they had begun an intimate letter correspondence even before the McKeages left Hooper and, being the same age, found that they had much in common. Lula could not wait to meet her.

As the train pulled into the Denver station, Lula and her parents were waiting on the platform straining to see each passenger as they disembarked. Although Eva and Nettie had not seen each other in many years, recognition was almost instantaneous, and they rushed to each other and hugged and kissed warmly. The others were more restrained. Blossom stood cautiously beside her two younger brothers, Rob and Charlie, wondering how she should react. She was by nature a reserved person, not given to hugging and kissing. But, when she saw a pretty blond girl running toward her, she felt her inhibitions relaxing and soon found herself hugging her cousin Lula. The two girls talked all the way to the Mooks' home, although it was mostly Lula talking and Blossom listening. There were so many things that Lula wanted to show her cousin in Denver, but at the top of the list was "her" handsome young medical student. Since this was Friday, that day would come soon.

Bruce Leslie stood at the door, welcoming each young lady by name as they filed into his classroom. When Lula and her cousin reached the front of the line, he found himself looking down at a face he had not seen before. Unlike Lula, she did not have the flashy beauty that made all the boys' heads turn, but a subtle, deep beauty that was not lost on Bruce. Her skin was smooth and creamy and made the perfect setting for her soft brown eyes, which reflected modesty, if not shyness. She had full and perfectly shaped lips that expressed a serious nature, but at the same time had the faint hint of a perpetual smile. Her abundant auburn hair was pulled back from her face and piled high in the back with a neat bun. In contrast to her cousin's frilly dress, Blossom wore a simple brown suit with black trim, the hem of which stopped just above her ankles. Her white blouse had a high lace collar that encircled her neck as though it were a vase supporting a delicate bouquet.

The two young people stood facing each other for a moment, both a bit ill at ease, waiting for Lula to make the introductions, which she hastened to do. She sidled up beside Bruce, as close as propriety would allow, looked up at him with her big blue eyes, and said, "Bruce, I would like you to meet my cousin, Blossom McKeage, from Leadville. She will be staying with us for the summer."

"Pleased to meet you, Blossom," he responded with a courteous smile.

"And you," Blossom replied in a quiet voice, as she returned a faint smile. She did not make eye contact, but demurely offered her right hand.

Bruce took her hand in both of his and held it for a moment, as was his custom when he wished to express a warm greeting. With her dainty hand in his two large but gentle ones, Blossom suddenly felt a tingling sensation rush through her entire body. Then, for the first time, she looked up into his kind hazel eyes, at which point a dreadful thing happened—she blushed.

Blossom hated it when she blushed. Her whole face would turn crimson, which she could tell by the warmth, and she was certain that it made her appear quite unattractive. Furthermore, it exposed her inner emotions. But, if Bruce noticed, he did not reveal it. In fact, his eyes had already lifted to the next woman in line. Lula grabbed her cousin's arm and helped her find a seat, then left for her own classroom.

During his lesson that day, Bruce found himself frequently looking over at the new face in the class. There was something different about her. She seemed genuinely interested in what he had to say.

It wasn't that the others didn't pay attention, but he often wondered if they were doing it just out of courtesy. In any case, he was rather pleased when Blossom returned the following Sunday. Since Lula had her own class to teach, her cousin began coming to the young ladies' class by herself. After the class, Bruce and Blossom would talk while they waited for Lula to join them. He found their conversations to be unusually pleasant. Instead of talking about the latest gossip in town, she preferred to discuss the topic of the day's lesson and often asked questions that he found quite searching.

As the warm days of summer glided by, Bruce began to allow himself a little more time for social life with the young folks in the church. Since he was now in his clinical rotations at the medical school, there was less demand for hitting the books, and he felt that he could afford to attend picnics on Sunday afternoons and other weekend activities. Of course, Lula and Blossom were always part of these group outings. Bruce enjoyed talking with both of them, although he began to wish that he and Blossom could have some time alone for their more serious talks. And he occasionally got his wish, when other young men would talk Lula into going with them for a boat ride or other venture. Those moments together in the summer of 1900 were the beginning of a special bonding for the two young people.

As the summer was coming to an end and Blossom prepared to return to Leadville, the Mooks hosted a gala dinner party at their home in her honor. It was destined to be the social event of the season, with everyone who was anyone being on the invitation list. Bruce received his invitation with mixed emotions. He was never comfortable at such high society affairs, and the only suit he had was threadbare. Nevertheless, he was grateful to have one last opportunity to see Blossom before she left. When he arrived at the Mook home that Saturday evening, it seemed that every light in the house was on. Colorful Japanese lanterns illuminated the wraparound porch and backyard. A large crowd already filled the house and yard, talking and laughing in loud voices in order to be heard over all the others who were talking and laughing in loud voices. Lula spotted him at the front door and rushed to his side. He was happy to see a familiar face but couldn't keep from looking around the room for another face—and then he saw her.

Blossom had a new dress for the occasion. It was made of pink lawn with a tiny white figurine print. It had a yoke with a ruffle around it and a long skirt that reached just above the floor. Bruce was stunned by her elegance and beauty and suddenly felt that he was wearing blinders, as he could see no one else in the room.

He spent what he hoped was an appropriate amount of time with Lula and then excused himself, which wasn't too hard, since she was always surrounded by a circle of attentive young men. He made his way to Blossom, who was just as thankful to be rescued by him from a boring conversation as he was to rescue her. They quietly slipped out of the house and into the backyard, where they found a bench under a distant Japanese lantern, away from the view of most of the partygoers. There they spent the rest of the evening, talking about many things. As the guests began to depart, and they too knew that they must say goodbye, they both wondered what the other was thinking and if they would ever meet again.

As Bruce entered his final semester of medical school, he began thinking about where he would go to set up his practice. He had offers in Denver, but there were already so many doctors there, and he really wanted to get back closer to home. He prayed about it every day, and one day the answer truly seemed to fall from heaven. The dean of the school held a meeting with the senior students to discuss their futures and announced that he had received a letter from a Mr. A. D. Kennedy, who was a banker in a small town in Indian Territory called Okmulgee. They needed a doctor, and the banker indicated that he was particularly interested in recruiting a young homeopath physician. A long silence followed the Dean's announcement, as the students seemed to have no interest in such a remote place, which most of them had never heard of. During the interlude, Bruce did some quick thinking and finally raised his hand and broke the silence.

"Well, sir, I guess I'm your man. I spent some time in Okmulgee a number of years ago and always thought I might go back there someday."

And so it was that Mr. Kennedy of Okmulgee received a letter from the dean of the Denver Homeopathic Medical College, informing him of the impending arrival that summer of one Dr. S. B. Leslie.

On a sunny day in June of 1902, there was an air of excitement as the graduating seniors donned their caps and gowns in preparation for the commencement exercises. Despite all the courses he had taken over the years, this would be Bruce's first participation in a formal graduation program, and he could not suppress a sense of pride as he carefully placed the mortarboard on his head with the tassel hanging on his right. The gown was black satin and had a white collar with a white bowtie. And he was sporting something new—a well-trimmed mustache, which he thought he might need to make him look older when he started his practice in Okmulgee, although it would not last long.

Bruce's only regret was that his mother could not be there to share this moment with him. But he was thankful to have his cousins, Elmer and Lester. Lula and her parents were also in attendance, along with many others from the Tabernacle, as well as Bruce's first landlady, Sheriff Jones and his wife, and, of course, Dr. Burr. They all posed for pictures, and Bruce promised Lula that he would write to her, and she cried, and then it was all over.

It had been eight years since he first arrived in Denver with no idea what the future held for him. And now he was leaving as a doctor, with a small town in Indian Territory waiting for him to start his new life. He had met many special people along the way, whose friendships he knew he would cherish for the rest of his life. But there was one person who held a special place in his thoughts, and he wondered if he would ever see her again. The one thing he did know for certain was that he had been blessed during these past years beyond his wildest dreams. And so, as his train pulled out of the Denver station, Bruce closed his eyes and said a prayer of profound thanks.

CHAPTER 7

Okmulgee
1902–1907

THE GRATING CLATTER OF AN ALARM CLOCK shattered the peaceful silence of the early morning, and a hand reached out from beneath a pile of blankets to silence it. Dr. Bruce Leslie rolled over and sighed. He had been up much of the night delivering a baby, who seemed to be in no hurry to enter the world, and now his body craved sleep. His head sank back into the warm hollow of his pillow, as the cobwebs began to clear from his waking mind. Since arriving in Okmulgee six months ago, he had been at the beck and call of his patients every day of the week, night and day. But, despite his chronic lack of sleep, which had become the norm, he loved what he was doing and always looked forward to the challenges and opportunities of a new day. And, as his mind began to focus, he remembered that this was to be a very special day.

His small room was cold and dark, illuminated only by a shaft of pale moonlight coming through a single window that was rimmed in frost. Going from the warmth of his bed to the chill of the room was a momentary shock to his system, and he swung his arms briskly back and forth to get his circulation going and to generate some body heat. He moved gingerly into his morning routine, first making up his bed by pulling the sheet and blankets tightly and neatly over the mattress and pillow. He knew that no one was likely to see inside his bedroom, but he maintained that it was important for a person to be neat and orderly in all their ways. He next slipped into a pair of cold boots and donned an overcoat that hung on a nail beside the back door. With that fortification, he opened the door and stepped out into the darkness and the frigid morning air. He looked up at the moon and the stars that twinkled in the firmament and could not help but wonder, as he had done so often, at the mystery of it all—not so much a mystery, perhaps, he reminded himself, as a reassurance.

The frozen brown grass—mostly weeds, actually—crunched beneath his boots as he walked across the backyard, adding to the sense of the morning chill. During the last half of the nineteenth century, indoor plumbing had become increasingly common, and by the turn of the century most of the finer homes were designed with indoor bathrooms. But the house in which Bruce resided was neither new nor fine, and so he made his way to the outdoor privy.

On his way back to the house, he picked up an armload of kindling from a stack beside the back door and placed it in a cast-iron stove in his room. With the help of pages from yesterday's newspaper, he started a fire and set a metal pitcher of water atop the stove. Keeping his coat and boots on for warmth while he waited for the fire to heat the room, he sat down on a straight wooden chair beside the stove and opened his Bible.

It was the one his father had given him from his deathbed when Bruce was still a young boy, and holding it never failed to bring back those memories. It had been his companion ever since that poignant time, and it served as a reminder of his heritage—familial and spiritual. He had always tried to find time for daily scripture reading, but it had not been easy during his medical school days. Now, with his life taking on the semblance of a routine, he had made it a practice to begin each day by reading one chapter. He preferred the New Testament and would proceed methodically from Matthew to Revelation, chapter by chapter. Before starting over again with Matthew, he would read a book from the Old Testament. There were parts of the Old Testament that he found hard to understand—how to rationalize the wars and killings with a God of love and mercy. But there were many books among those ancient texts in which he found great comfort, especially Psalms and Proverbs. He also enjoyed reading some of the prophets and many of the old stories like Job and, in particular, Ruth. He was well into the current cycle of his New Testament reading, and this morning he read the first chapter in the book of James: "Be ye doers of the word and not hearers only." He smiled at the old familiar words. He knew them by heart, and that verse would always be among his favorites.

After reading the chapter and reflecting on its meaning, he closed his eyes for his morning prayer. He always began with thanksgiving for all his blessings—good health, an education, an opportunity to serve in this community, and all the promises that lay before him. Then he offered prayers of intercession for his loved ones. He prayed for his widowed mother back in Arkansas, and for his two half-sisters, Ona and Ollie, although he barely knew them. And he prayed for his brother Eb, who was still living in Texas, and for his sister Floy, who had married and moved to South Dakota, and for all his aunts, uncles, and cousins, wherever they might be. Finally, he prayed for guidance, that his actions, his words, and his thoughts in the day that lay ahead might be in accordance with God's wishes. This was how he began the day—with scripture reading and prayer—and it was how he would start every day for the remainder of his life.

The water was beginning to boil on the stove as he opened his eyes from praying. He used a portion of it to make his coffee and poured some into a pan of oats, which he stirred until they were edible. He stayed close to the warmth of the stove as he ate his breakfast, sipped his coffee, and read the remainder of yesterday's newspaper. Then he poured the last of the hot water into an enamel basin and prepared to shave. He dipped his brush in the hot water and swished it around in his shaving mug until the lather foamed to the top. He brushed the warm suds on his face and then swiped his straight razor back-and-forth several times on a leather strop. The mustache that he had sported during graduation from medical school had long since disappeared. Although he had looked quite dapper in it, he just didn't feel it was him, and for the rest of his life he would be clean-shaven. After combing his hair, he put on his cleanest white shirt, his only suit, and one of the two ties he owned. He was now ready to meet the new day.

He had been renting two rooms—the one in which he lived and an adjacent room that served as a clinic for seeing his patients. The front foyer of the house connected to the clinic room and served as a waiting area, where there would typically be several patients waiting by this time of the morning. But, on this particular day, there was no one in sight, and his clinic was practically bare. Where just recently he had his desk and all the furnishings for patient care, he now stood in the silence of the empty room—a room that brought back a host of memories and emotions. Although he had been practicing medicine for only six months, he had witnessed the full range of human drama in that room, from announcing the joyful news to young parents that their infant child was healthy and normal to sharing the heartbreaking reality with an elderly couple that nothing more could be done.

The memories swirled around him as he paused for a moment and reflected on all that had happened during the past six months.

❦

The train ride out of Denver had been a true pleasure for the young medical school graduate—much more so than years before, when he had been traveling in the opposite direction. Then his heart had been heavy with the thought of leaving behind his family and friends and the only life he had ever known. And he had felt the uneasiness of conflicting emotions—the exhilaration of facing new adventures and opportunities and yet the uncertainty of what lay ahead in his life and where it would take him. But eight years later, as he was leaving Denver, he had looked out the train window at the passing landscape and felt a great sense of Providence at the clear and promising road ahead. It was as though the clouds had parted to reveal blue sky for as far as the eye could see and warm sunshine to brighten the path that his life was about to take. He had marveled, once again, at how events in our lives—some of which seem so dark at the time—can radically alter the course of our life and send us off in new directions that we could never have imagined. And, always mindful of the source of his blessings, he had frequently closed his eyes during the long train ride to offer thanks.

The train had rumbled all night through the farmlands of Kansas, and the sun was rising as it crossed the border into Indian Territory. By noon, it was entering the Tulsa station, pulling in alongside trains from all over the country. He had purchased a ticket from Denver to Sapulpa, which was about thirty miles from Okmulgee, because the agent in Denver thought the Frisco line was not yet running to Okmulgee. But, when he arrived in Tulsa, he found that passenger trains were indeed operating through to Okmulgee. And so, after a layover until midafternoon, he departed on the final leg of his journey, and, as the sun was beginning to set, the train pulled in to the small Okmulgee station.

As he stood on the station platform, wondering what he should do next, a dignified, elderly gentleman walked up to him and inquired if he was Dr. Leslie. Hearing his new title momentarily took him aback, but he confirmed his identity and found himself shaking the hand of Mr. A. D. Kennedy, the banker who had helped bring him to Okmulgee. He welcomed Bruce warmly and asked if he would come to his home for dinner. Although he was exhausted from the many hours of traveling, he felt he could not decline—and, besides, he was famished. When they arrived at the Kennedy home, Bruce was introduced to Mrs. Kennedy and another couple, Mr. and Mrs. Joe C. Trent, who he learned had also been instrumental in bringing him to Okmulgee. They were all gracious and welcoming, but Bruce took a special liking to Mr. Kennedy, whom everyone seemed to affectionately call Father Kennedy.

It was a delicious meal and a pleasant evening, but knowing Bruce had to be tired from his long journey, they mercifully made it a short evening. The Trents took him in their buggy to the hotel, where he slept soundly for the first time in many hours.

The following morning, Bruce stepped out of his hotel and looked around at his new hometown, seeing it in the full light of day for the first time since leaving it many years before. It hadn't changed a great deal. The Creek Council House still occupied the center of the town square, surrounded by a wide lawn and a stone wall. All the streets were dirt, muddy from a recent rain. There were wooden sidewalks in front of the buildings around the square, and Bruce later noted with amusement that they often "heaved and tossed" because hogs, which frequently roamed free, would get under the boards and rub against them to scratch their backs.

He found a diner on the square and, walking in, was greeted by the hearty aroma of bacon and coffee. In the corner, a group of men sat around a table, seemingly engrossed in an intense conversation. A middle-aged woman, wearing an apron and a net around her hair, stood behind the counter and gave the newcomer a big smile.

"Morning, sugar," she called out. Bruce looked behind him to see who she might be talking to and concluded that it must be him. He smiled and nodded and walked over to a stool at the counter.

"What can I get for you, sugar?" She certainly had a way of making a fellow feel welcome, he thought. The menu, written in chalk on a black board, offered a special of *Bacon, eggs, toast, and coffee 25¢*. He felt the coins in his pocket and questioned whether he should be so extravagant. But it was the first day in his new hometown and he wanted to make a good impression on the town folk, so he decided to splurge and ordered the special.

"You the new doctor?" the waitress asked as she poured his coffee. Bruce couldn't help but smile at how fast news seemed to spread in a small town.

"Yes ma'am, I guess I am that," he responded.

The waitress was not the only one in the diner whose attention was drawn to the newcomer. The conversation had ceased over in the corner and all eyes were directed toward the counter. One of the men stood up and walked over to Bruce.

"You the new doc?" he was asked, for the second time in as many minutes.

"Yes sir. Bruce Leslie's the name," he replied as he extended his hand.

"Pleased to meet you, Dr. Leslie, and welcome to Okmulgee," he said as they shook hands. "I'm George King. Me and the boys would be honored to have you come join us."

Bruce gratefully accepted the invitation and carried his half-empty coffee mug over to meet the "boys," most of whom were of retirement age. They were all white, except for one who seemed to have some Native American features. For the next few minutes, the conversation focused on the young doctor as he answered their questions about his background. Then it shifted back to what the men had been discussing previously, which was the topic on everyone's mind—statehood.

It was not just a question of statehood, they explained to Bruce. Most people, with notable exceptions, agreed that that was a good idea. The main issue that drove the debates was whether there should be one state or two. The land runs of the 1890s had created a section in the western half of the territory that became known as Oklahoma Territory, while the eastern half, controlled by five Indian Nations, continued to be called Indian Territory. It was actually the creation of Oklahoma Territory that had started the quest for statehood, and it was primarily the Native Americans who argued for separate states. The question had become a major issue in Washington, where President Roosevelt favored a single state, while Vice-President Taft leaned toward two. Of course, there were many other issues related to statehood, including Indian rights, civil rights, women's suffrage, prohibition, mining regulations, and delineation of counties, all of which, Bruce soon learned, provided fodder for countless hours of heated debate, most of which he studiously avoided.

After breakfast, he walked a few blocks from the town square to a white frame structure known as the Arlington House, which had been recommended to him the night before by Mr. Kennedy. He was met at the front door by the landlady, who confirmed that two rooms were available for rent on the first floor, just off a large foyer with stairs that went up to the second floor. She took him into a sparsely furnished room with a well-worn black leather couch and two oak chairs beside a window. Although it was not particularly impressive, Bruce could see the possibilities for this room as his medical office and clinic. A second room opened off the first, and contained a single bed, a small oak dresser, and a cast-iron stove, with a door that led to the backyard. The two rooms were all he would need to start his practice and have a place to live, and he proceeded to work out the financial arrangements with his new landlady.

His next stop was back downtown to the bank, where he was scheduled to meet Father Kennedy at 10 a.m. The elderly gentleman greeted him warmly and asked if his hotel accommodations had been satisfactory. Bruce assured him that they were and told him how the morning had gone thus far. They then walked down the hall and through a door with LOAN OFFICE inscribed on the frosted window. Mr. Kennedy introduced Bruce to the loan officer, who he promised would take good care of him. When the two were alone and had completed their pleasantries, the loan officer asked the young doctor what he could do for him. Bruce suddenly felt rather ill at ease, having never before asked anyone for money. But he did need a loan to start his practice and rather timidly asked if $100 might be possible. The banker smiled and said that could certainly be arranged. Before leaving the bank, Bruce opened an account and withdrew $10 from the teller. And so, as he walked out of the bank into the morning sunshine, young Dr. Leslie now had a place to live, a place to practice, and money in the bank and in his pocket.

On his way back to the hotel to pick up his belongings, he stopped off at the general store for a few supplies. He introduced himself to the young man behind the counter, who appeared to be one of the indigenous people in his early twenties. Bruce was interested to learn that the name of his new acquaintance was Amos McIntosh, which brought back memories of the family he had met on his first journey into the territory. Amos explained that he was related to the McIntoshes of Muskogee and that all of his people had come from Georgia in the previous century. As the conversation warmed up, something told the two young men that they were destined to become good friends, a feeling that the decades ahead would bear out. Bruce picked up a loaf of bread and some apples and then went over to the office supply section and selected a cloth-bound ledger, with the word "Journal" across the front cover. It was in this book that he would soon begin to record the patients that he would be caring for over the next half century.

When he arrived back at his new quarters, he was surprised to find two people waiting for him in the foyer. Mrs. Kennedy had brought her daughter, Leonida, who had awakened that morning with an earache. Bruce took them into his empty "clinic" and performed an examination with the instruments he had in his black leather bag. He found that the young lady had otitis media, or an ear infection, a condition with which he had become quite familiar during his medical school days and on which he would one day publish a paper in a medical journal. He wrote out a prescription to be filled at the local apothecary and instructed Leonida on its use. Mrs. Kennedy and her daughter—his first patient—were obviously very impressed with the professionalism and skill of the new young doctor and would soon share their opinion with friends and neighbors. And thus began the medical practice of Dr. Samuel Brewster Leslie.

Despite the endorsement by his first patient, the practice did not take off immediately, which gave him the time he needed to set up his office. On his second full day in town, he stood in the sparsely furnished room that was to become the clinic and made a mental note of the additional items he would need. The day before, he had noticed a store that sold used furniture, and he decided to make that his first stop of the day. There he found a tall oak secretary with glassed-in shelves on the top and a door that opened from below to make a desk with many cubbyholes in the back. He decided that this would serve well as both his desk and a place to store his medications while taking up minimal floor space. Moreover, the price was right. He also picked out a captain's chair to go with it, a glass-front bookcase to store all the used books he had acquired in medical school, and a long, narrow table on which he would examine his patients. The total for all the items came to $17, and he made the payment and arranged for shipment to his office that afternoon.

His next stop was the apothecary, where he purchased several bottles of the basic medications he would be prescribing. These included carbolic acid, calomel, iodine, compound cathartic pills, sulfur, glycothymaline, No. 1 rectal suppositories, Scott's Emulsion, peroxide of hydrogen, and a bottle of sugar pills for the children and the occasional placebo effect. Finally, he went to the local printer, where he ordered a sign for his office. He had considered several variations of his name and tried them out on the inside cover of his ledger but decided that the initials would appear the most distinguished and professional. And so the sign on his clinic door read "Dr. S. B. Leslie." For the remainder of his life, he would be known by most people as Dr. Leslie, while his closer acquaintances called him S. B., and only the most intimate used the name Bruce.

So now he was set to launch his practice. In Denver he had bought the few instruments he would need for diagnoses and treatments, which he kept in his black bag. But physicians in those days did not depend heavily on technology, especially not for diagnosing disease. They relied much more on a careful history, their finely honed skills of visual and auditory observation, and their senses of touch and smell. In years to come, it was said that Dr. Leslie could often make the diagnosis of a patient simply by walking into their home and smelling the telltale odor of the disease.

There was one telephone in the foyer of Arlington House for use by all the boarders where S. B. lived and worked. It was customary for whoever was closest to the phone to answer it and then find the person for whom the call was intended. In time, however, it became obvious that most of the calls were for the doctor, especially those in the wee hours of the night, and so he would usually pick up the phone whenever he was home. But many of his patients did not yet have a telephone, which was just coming into common use at the turn of the century, and he would often find them in the morning, biding their time on the black leather couch that he had placed in the foyer, which served as a waiting room. After office hours and at any time of the night, they would come around to the back of the house and knock on the door to his sleeping quarters. And he would always bring them in to take care of their needs or go with them to the home where a patient required his services.

Although most of the patients were seen in his clinic, Dr. Leslie also made several house calls every day of the week and at any hour of the night. The mode of transportation with which he began his practice was his two feet. If the home was close enough, he would walk to it. For country calls, he would rent a saddle horse from the livery stable. It would only be later, when he felt that he could afford it, that he bought his own horse, and later still before he would travel with his horse and buggy.

Like most physicians of his day—a time well before the age of specialization—Dr. Leslie would see in his practice the full range of human joy and suffering. He was there to stand beside young couples at the time of birth, to help ease his little patients into the world and nurse them through their infancy, to dress the wounds of his patients, to help them through their diseases and afflictions, to extend their lives as much as possible, and to be there to ease their final days when he had no more to offer. All these encounters he recorded in his ledgers.

Individual patient records were not commonly used in those days, and the electronic medical records of today could not even have been imagined. In his ledger, beneath the day's date, he would write a brief description of the patients he had seen that day. Beginning with the name of the patient or relative in the left-hand column ("Mrs. Chonleys," "Mr. King," "Mr. Dodd," "Alois Alt," "Mr. Scott for Mother," and so on), he would then note their condition, his thoughts, and a plan for their treatment. In the far right-hand column, he would enter the fee. In the early days, this was fifty cents for most visits and a dollar or two for more complex cases and house calls. Many patients could not even afford that, and he would accept whatever they had to offer—produce from their farm, credit in their store, a haircut, or anything they had. On one occasion, a minister who was in town for a series of lectures and was bothered by "throat trouble" paid him with a life membership in the American Sunday League. And then there were those who had nothing to give. But he never turned anyone away.

There were two older doctors in Okmulgee when S. B. first arrived, Dr. Hensley and Dr. Gardner, and he would occasionally see one of their patients when they were away, as they would do for him. For the most part, however, Dr. Leslie was on call 24/7, taking whatever cases came his way. The work was challenging and exhausting, but the young doctor found it exhilarating—he had found his purpose in life and thanked God every day for the opportunity to serve others.

∽ ҉

Those first six months of his practice had gone by quickly. Now, as he stood in his empty clinic on that special morning, bathed in the memories of all the drama he had witnessed in his nascent medical practice, he hoped that he was not moving too fast. And yet, he felt a sense of comforting reassurance in the thought that this day was the beginning of the next chapter in his career and in his life.

Bruce was true to his Scottish heritage in his practice of thrift. Aside from sending some of his money home each month to his mother in Arkansas, he saved every penny he could, allowing himself only the most basic needs. As a result, he had enough in his savings account after six months to rent a proper medical office in the new Bank of Commerce building, a red-brick two-story structure just off the town square. His office was on the second floor above Mr. Kennedy's bank, and had a large window facing the street on which was inscribed "Dr S. B. Leslie." A wide tiled staircase led from the sidewalk below to a small landing that served several offices on that floor. The door to his office opened into the waiting room, where he had placed the black leather couch and one of the oak chairs that he purchased from his landlady. The second and larger of the two rooms was his office and clinic. Positioned near the window was the oak secretary, which served as both his desk and a pharmacy for his medicine bottles behind the glassed-in front. He used his oak captain's chair at his desk and placed the other oak chair close by for his patients. To the right of this was the glass-fronted case containing all his medical books, over which hung his diploma from medical school, and on the other side of the room was the table on which he examined his patients.

He had planned it all out carefully and could see it in his mind as he stepped out of his old quarters into the frigid January air. The year was 1903, and he could not help but wonder what it might hold in store for him. This time last year, he was still a medical student, and now he was an established physician on his way to the first day in his impressive new office.

He didn't make appointments in those days—patients just came when they had a need—and he wondered if anyone would be waiting for him when he arrived. Of course, they would have to be waiting on the landing, since the door to the waiting room was locked. But, upon ascending the shiny tile stairs to the second floor, he found the landing empty and felt a bit disappointed to be entering his new office all alone on this first day. For such a special occasion, he felt like he should be sharing it with someone. But he laughed at his foolishness as he reached for the door knob and began to insert his key. For a moment, however, his mood changed to one of mild concern when he realized that the door was not locked. And what he discovered upon entering his waiting room left him speechless.

The room was packed shoulder-to-shoulder with people who suddenly shouted as one, "Hip hip hooray! Hip hip hooray!" and then began laughing and offering the young doctor their hands in congratulations. It seemed that everyone in the town was there—all the Kennedys and the Trent family, his landlady and his good friend Amos McIntosh, and many of his patients whom he had treated during those first six months. After everyone had had a chance to shake the doctor's hand and wish him well, Father Kennedy asked for their attention.

"Bruce—or, I should say, Dr. Leslie," he began with a smile, as the group shared a friendly chuckle at his correction. "You have surely won the hearts and respect of all of us in Okmulgee during your brief time in our midst. We have come to know that we can count on you, day or night, to be there whenever one of us is in need. You have shown skill and knowledge, professionalism and compassion as you treated our wounds and healed our infirmities. I know that I speak for everyone in saying how pleased and proud we are to have you as a valued member of our community. This is a fine clinic that you have established and, on behalf of all of us, I congratulate you and wish you many years of successful practice within these walls."

Again, there was shouting and clapping and "hooraying" as everyone put an exclamation mark on Father Kennedy's kind words. Bruce felt himself choking up a bit at all the expressions of thoughtfulness, especially when Father Kennedy approached him with his big hand outstretched. Bruce had always made a point of looking people directly in the eye, and, as he did so now, his emotions once again changed from lightheartedness to concern. His benefactor must have wondered when he saw the expression on the young man's face change from a smile to a bit of a frown. But he just assumed it was the stress of the excitement, and neither man said anything about it. For the young doctor, however, it would be a moment that he would always remember as the beginning of one of the most challenging times in his practice of medicine.

What S. B. had seen when he looked into the eyes of Father Kennedy was a faint yellowish discoloration to the whites of his eyes. He knew that this could mean a serious problem in the liver—hepatitis or even cancer. He hoped that he had been mistaken but knew that he had to take a closer look and wondered how he should approach the kindly gentleman who had become like a father to him.

One of the first things that Bruce had done after arriving in Okmulgee, six months ago, was to visit the Methodist Church, which he had first attended many years before when he came to the town as a traveling salesman of fruit trees. They had a new pastor now, and Bruce liked him as much as he had the previous one. Furthermore, the Kennedys were members of the congregation, and that was enough to convince

Bruce that this was where he wanted to establish his membership—one that he would retain for the remainder of his life. So, as he thought about what he had seen in Father Kennedy's eyes, he felt that Sunday morning would afford a good chance to get a closer look at the patriarch and decide if further action was warranted.

As he walked to church that Sunday morning, there was a frosting of snow on the ground from the night before, and he pulled the collar of his overcoat more tightly around his neck. He wondered if the chill he felt was from the weather or from his concern as to what he might encounter when he saw Father Kennedy. The warmth inside the church lifted his spirits a bit, as did the music and the scripture readings and the sermon. He sat toward the back of the sanctuary, as was his custom, and waited in the narthex after the service as the other parishioners filed out and congregated in small groups to chat. Bruce made his way over to the Kennedy family, who were engaged in a lively conversation with friends. He tried to reflect the casual mirth of the group as he stepped into their circle, but his countenance suddenly fell when Father Kennedy turned toward him. The elderly gentleman must have wondered at the expression on the young doctor's face and why he was staring at him so intently. And Bruce was momentarily lost for words, as he looked at the undeniable yellow discoloration in his friend's eyes and realized that his greatest fear was confirmed. The two made small talk for a moment, about the weather and the sermon, and then S. B. asked him when he had last had a medical checkup. Mr. Kennedy now began to put two and two together and admitted to the doctor that it had been some time and that he had, in fact, been feeling a bit "puny" lately. And so it was agreed that they would meet the following morning in Dr. Leslie's office.

He was just leaving the boarding house for his office the next morning when the phone in the foyer rang and Bruce picked it up to hear the voice of Mrs. Kennedy. She sounded concerned and said that Mr. Kennedy did not want to get out of bed. She suspected it was just a cold from the inclement weather but wondered if the doctor could stop by the house sometime during the day. He felt a chill go through his body and prayed that it was just a cold, although he feared it was something far worse. He told Mrs. Kennedy that he would come right over, picked up his black bag, and headed out into the snowy morning—and the first great challenge of his medical career.

The Kennedy home was warmer than S. B. was accustomed to, and he slipped off his overcoat as he stepped into the Kennedys' bedroom. He was startled to see how his patient's condition had changed in just one day. Father Kennedy's face was moist with perspiration and, through the glistening film, Bruce could now see the telltale sign of yellow in his skin as well as his eyes. He knew this to be jaundice and that it most likely represented serious liver disease. His patient's forehead was not only yellow but hot with fever, and his pulse was rapid and a bit weak. He palpated the abdomen, expecting to feel an enlarged liver, but found nothing out of the ordinary other than a little tenderness. He concluded that there must be an inflammation of the liver, which he hoped would reverse with time, and gave Mr. Kennedy some tonics to make him feel better until he got over the worst of his condition.

He stopped by the Kennedys' on his way home from the office that evening and was encouraged to find his patient sitting up and feeling and looking a bit better. He advised him to continue the tonics and promised that he would stop by each day but urged them to call if there were any changes. That night he included Father Kennedy in his prayers, thanking God that he seemed to be responding to the treatment and beseeching that he continue on the road to recovery. But Bruce knew that God does not always answer our prayers the way we wish, and this would not be the last time that he would be reminded of the need to accept God's will and not our own. Sometime in the wee hours of the morning, the phone rang, and Dr. Leslie again found himself talking with Mrs. Kennedy. This time she sounded more distressed than ever and informed the doctor that her husband's fever seemed higher and that he was delirious. Bruce said he would be right there.

As he entered the bedroom, the smell of sickness accosted his nostrils and sent a chill of foreboding through his body. It was one of the smells that he would come to recognize all too well in the years ahead, but on this night he knew only that it was not an encouraging sign. Mr. Kennedy was lying in a pool of perspiration and, as his wife had feared, was in a state of delirium, not seeming to know where he was and thrashing about uncontrollably. He was burning up, and Bruce knew he had to get his temperature down quickly. He immediately went about applying cold compresses and gave him a sedative to relax him. As the dawn light began to shine through the bedroom window, Father Kennedy's temperature was coming down, and he looked around as though wondering where he was. Exhausted but relieved at his patient's improvement, Bruce had no choice but to go on to his office, where other patients would be waiting for his care. He promised he would return that evening or sooner if necessary.

As the weary young doctor entered the Kennedy home that evening, he was elated to find his patient sitting up and in his right mind. But he knew that much of the improvement was from the medications he was on and that the future was still gravely in doubt. And, sadly, his premonitions would be justified in the days and weeks that lay ahead. It would be a roller coaster of good days and bad, and the young Dr. Leslie would go through a rite of passage that all physicians must experience when they realize that their skills and knowledge are woefully inadequate. But Bruce took it harder than most. He literally wept some nights at his inability to help his dear friend and wondered what the townspeople must think of their doctor, who could not save one of their most beloved citizens. He sought consultation from the other doctors in town and from noted physicians nearby, but none had anything more to offer.

The day finally came when Bruce had to accept the fact that he could do nothing more and that the fate of his patient was in the hands of a higher power. He continued to pray but felt that his faith was waning, and he was beginning to prepare himself for the worst. One night, when his despair seemed to have reached its peak, he lay awake for hours, praying and trying to think what more he could do—what he might have missed. He had just drifted into a fitful sleep when the alarm went off. For once in his life, he did not want to face the day. It was not because of fatigue, but of fear—fear of what he would find when he returned to the Kennedy home.

Despite his negative feelings, he got up and dressed quickly. He skipped breakfast; eating was the last thing on his mind. During the night, he had had a feeling that Father Kennedy's situation was changing. But was it for the worse—was he about to leave this world—

or was he possibly getting better? He was afraid to learn the answer, but he trudged resolutely to his patient's house. When Mrs. Kennedy met him at the door, her countenance seemed a bit more cheerful than he had seen in quite some time. And as he entered the house, he thought the air had a slightly better aroma. He tried to suppress these seemingly positive indicators as just his overwhelming desire for good news. But when he stepped into the Kennedy bedroom he knew that his feelings were not just vain hope.

Father Kennedy was sitting up and actually had a faint smile on his sunken face. As Bruce walked closer to him, he could see that the yellow coloration was fading from his eyes and skin. He checked his patient's vital signs and found them to be strong. And, at that moment, Dr. Leslie knew that his patient was going to live. But then a frightening thing happened—Bruce realized that he was losing control of his emotions. He took a deep breath and attempted to explain in his most professional tone that he was very pleased with Mr. Kennedy's progress. The Kennedys, of course, were overjoyed and Mrs. Kennedy did not hold back her tears. Bruce said he needed to move on, but that he would stop back by in the evening. The truth is that he needed to leave the house while he still had a semblance of control.

As he stepped outside into the early morning sunshine, he felt the tears beginning to well up in his eyes. He looked around for a place where he would not be noticed, and there he let his emotions take over as he poured out his deepest gratitude in prayer. Dr. S. B. Leslie learned a lesson that day—one that he probably already knew but now would never doubt. It reminded him of a quotation he had learned in medical school that is attributed to an old French surgeon: "I treat, God heals."

⚭

The next several years flew by for Dr. Leslie. His practice grew rapidly as did his stature in the community. He brought many babies into the world, treated many wounds, set many fractures, cared for the full range of illnesses from colds to cancer. He rejoiced with his patients when the news was good and tried to always be by their side when nothing more could be done. And he never forgot that, whatever the outcome might be, it was ultimately in the hands of the one in whom he put his complete faith.

Despite his demanding schedule, Bruce made it a point to keep up on the latest news at home and around the world. As 1903 came to a close, he was fascinated to read that two men by the names of Orville and Wilbur Wright had flown a motor-powered flying machine on a beach called Kitty Hawk in North Carolina. He could not help but wonder where that would lead. The following February, he learned that the United States had acquired control of the Panama Canal Zone and would begin construction on the canal later that year. One minor news item that brought a smile to his face in the summer of 1904 was that something called an ice cream cone had been introduced at the St. Louis World's Fair. With time, that treat would become one of his weaknesses. But the news that most captivated everyone in those days were the events that would eventually lead to Oklahoma statehood.

As he had been informed by "the boys" in the diner shortly after his arrival in 1902, there was serious consideration given to creating two states out of Oklahoma Territory and Indian Territory. In 1905, the Sequoyah Convention met in Muskogee to draft a constitution for the separate state of Sequoyah. But the U.S. Congress ignored their act and instead passed the Oklahoma Enabling Act, which required joint statehood of the two territories. In March 1906, Congress passed the Five Tribes Act, which abolished tribal government, and in November of that year, a Constitutional Convention was held in Guthrie, Oklahoma, chaired by William "Alfalfa Bill" Murray, who would later become governor of Oklahoma. The constitution was approved by an overwhelming majority, and on November 17, 1907, President Roosevelt's signature made Oklahoma the forty-sixth state in the union. It was a time of celebration throughout the state and beyond. As for Bruce Leslie, he joined his Okmulgee townspeople in acknowledging the monumental event, but he worried about the effect it would have on his friends in the Indian nations and other minorities.

During those heady days in Oklahoma and around the world, major changes were also occurring in the life of Dr. Leslie. He had long been concerned about his mother and two step-sisters back in Arkansas and wanted to bring them to Okmulgee where he could take better care of them. But he was still living in the small quarters of his boarding house and lacked a suitable dwelling to accommodate the three women. He decided it was time that he had a home in keeping with the stature that he now enjoyed in the community—one to which he could bring his family.

He had been following the real estate market and consulting with a real estate agent whose office was adjacent to his, but they had been unable to find a suitable house for purchase. So Bruce eventually decided to buy a vacant lot and build a house. He decided on some prime property just a few blocks from downtown that was within walking distance from his office. It was an elevated lot that sloped down to the corner of East Third and Main Streets. There were currently no homes on the entire block, and Bruce purchased the corner lot as well as adjacent property, giving him possession of about one-fourth of the block. Then he turned his attention to building his home.

At the suggestion of his real estate agent, Bruce studied a Sears, Roebuck catalogue in which he found plans for a two-story white frame house that he thought would look good on his new property. In those days, it was possible to order a house from the catalogue and then have local builders assemble the component parts. The price of $725 was daunting, but, through years of hard work and frugality, he had saved nearly that amount and was able to cover the rest with a loan from the bank. And so, construction began on the house in which he would spend the remainder of his life.

The house faced East Third Street and was assigned the number 122. A wide, covered porch extended across the front of the house; a swing later hung from the porch ceiling. The front door had a cut-glass window and opened to a large foyer, from which heavy oak stairs wound up to the second floor. To the right of the foyer, a wide entrance with French doors led into the living room and then to the dining room at the back of the house. The latter two rooms were separated by dark red velvet curtains. The kitchen was just off the dining room, with a window that looked out over Main Street. Another wide porch extended across most of the back of the house and would become the main point of coming and going for the family in the years ahead. The back porch was also the place where bushels of vegetables and other payments-in-kind from the doctor's patients could be found at almost any time of the year.

At the top of the oak stairs, a long hallway opened onto four bedrooms and a single bathroom. In the years to come, as the family expanded, the latter room would become the busiest one in the house. At the end of the hallway was another room that was also among the most coveted, especially in the summer. It was the sleeping porch—a long, narrow room above the back porch that contained three beds, end-to-end, and was lined with large screened windows that allowed cool breezes to circulate during the warm seasons. On hot summer nights, long before the advent of air conditioning, it was the only place where a little relief could be found.

A white picket fence surrounded the backyard, which contained several shade trees and would one day be graced with flower beds, vegetable gardens, and a grape arbor. Further behind the backyard, Bruce built a barn where he would keep his horse and buggy and a cow—eventually, it would become the garage for his car. Adjacent to the barn was a chicken coop, which would provide eggs for the family and many fryers for Sunday meals.

And so he was finally able to write his mother and tell her that she and her two daughters could come to live with him in what was then one of the finest houses in Okmulgee. He met them at the train station and could barely contain his joy as he drove them in his horse and buggy to see their beautiful new home for the first time. The days and months that followed were among the happiest he had ever known. His mother immediately became the matriarch of the family and their homestead, bringing a sense of order into a man's world. Bruce loved coming home to her good cooking and to having the companionship of his two step-sisters. They both adored him and did all they could to ease the burdens of his demanding days. Life was good.

But the day soon came when Bruce realized that something was still missing in his life. In fact, he had been thinking about it for some time. He was, without question, one of the most eligible and desirable bachelors in Okmulgee and had met a number of young ladies, mostly at his church, who would like nothing more than to become Mrs. S. B. Leslie. But none of them seemed quite right; none shared his values and aspirations. Although it had been five years since leaving Denver, he had never forgotten a certain young woman he had met there. And so, late one night in the spring of 1908, he sat down and wrote a letter.

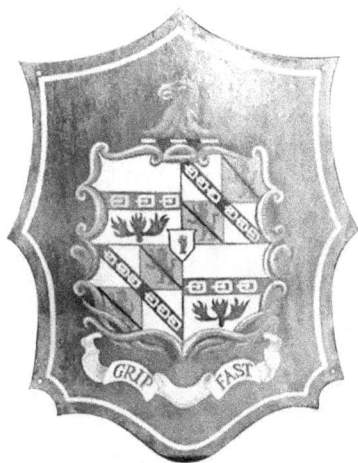

Clan Leslie coat of arms with motto "Grip Fast"
(Photographed in Castle Leslie, Glaslough, Ireland)

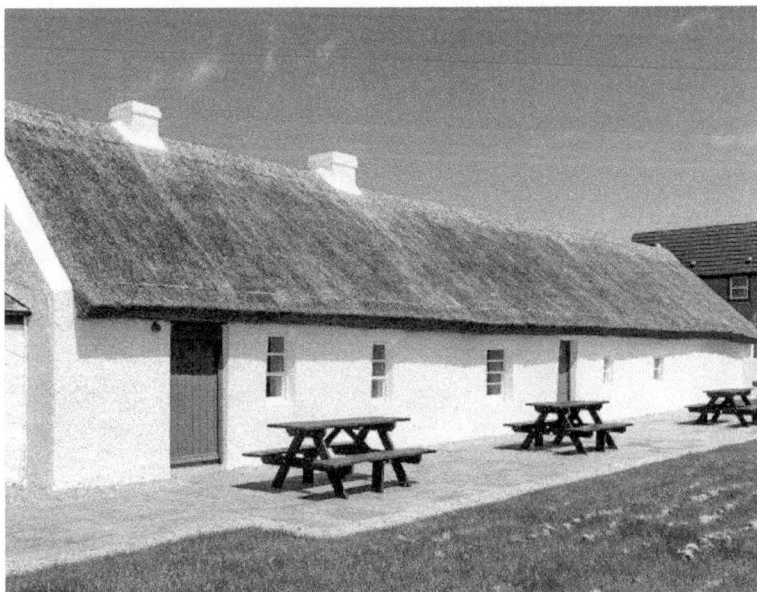

Eighteenth century cottage in Carrickfurgus, County Antrim, Ireland, near the
sites where the Leslie, Hutchinson, and Jackson family homes once stood

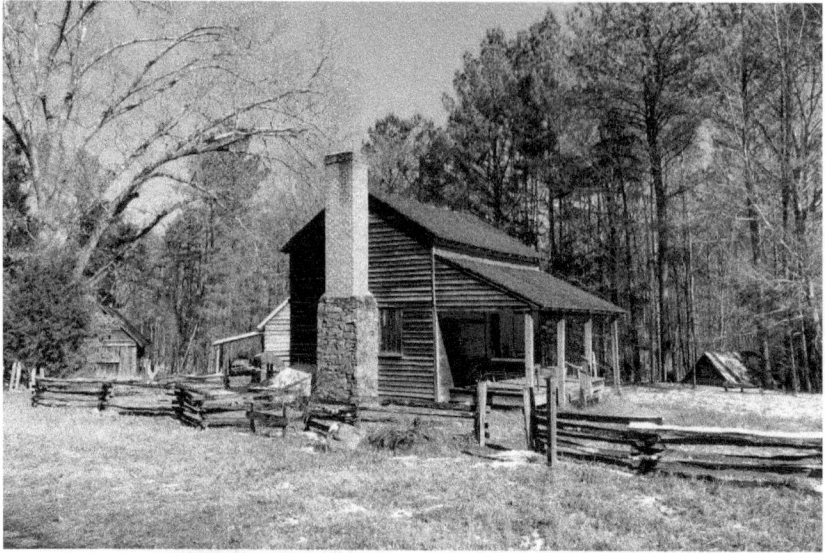

Pioneer farmhouse in Waxhaw, North Carolina, near the sites
where the farms of Samuel Leslie and his extended families
once stood (Picture taken at the Museum of the Waxhaws)

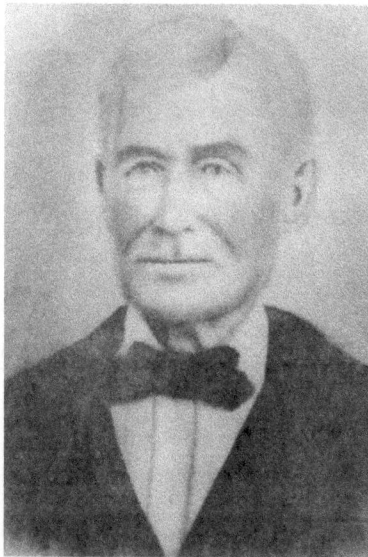

Samuel Leslie, after whom the town of Leslie, Arkansas, was named.
Grandfather of Bruce Leslie and great-great-grandfather of the author.

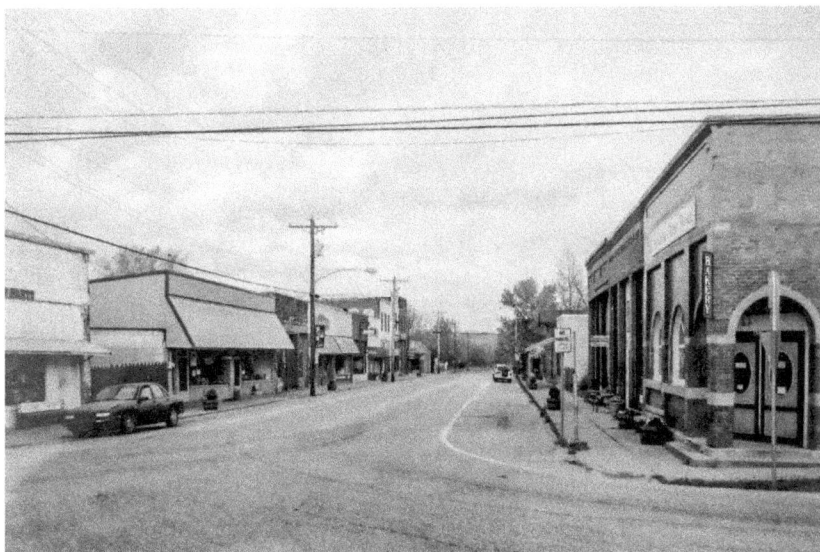

Leslie, Arkansas, in 2012
(Picture taken at corner of Main and Oak Streets)

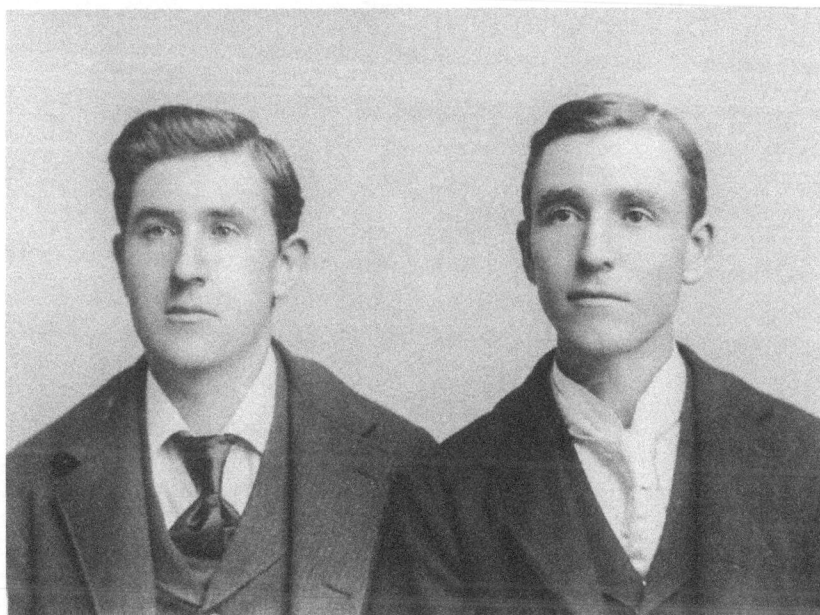

Bruce Leslie (right) and brother, Evans Green Leslie

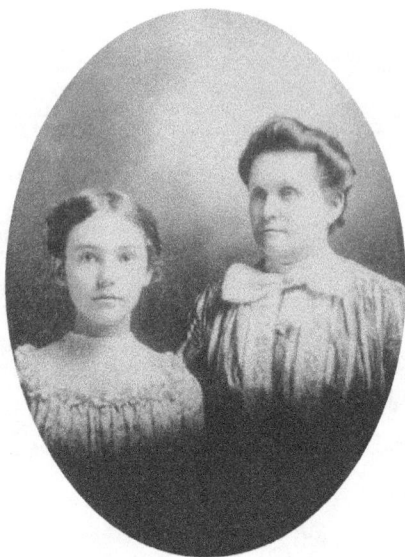

Bruce Leslie's mother, California "Callie" Jamima,
and his half-sister, Ollie

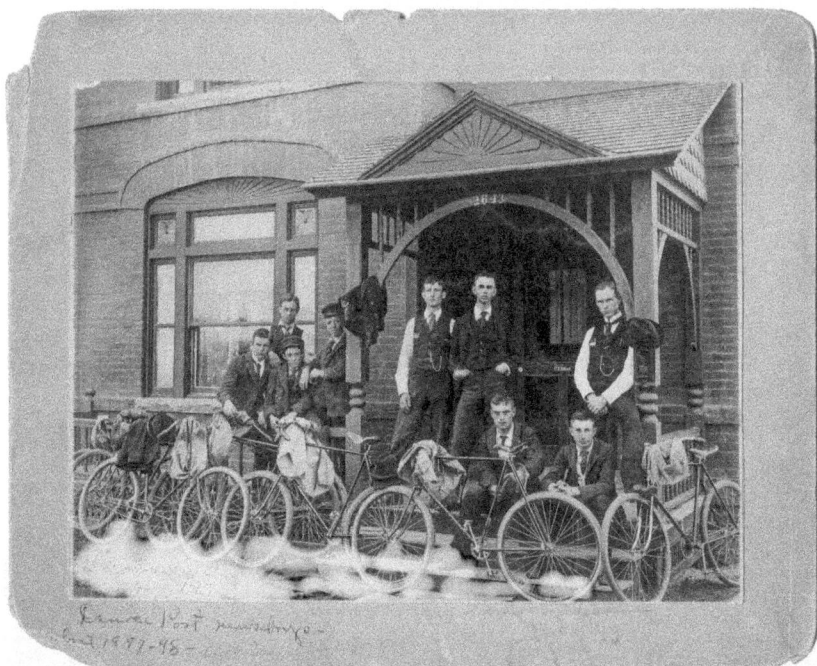

The Denver Carrier Club
Bruce Leslie is standing on steps at left; some carriers were working
their way through higher education and others vowed never to
darken the door of a school (can you pick the two groups?)

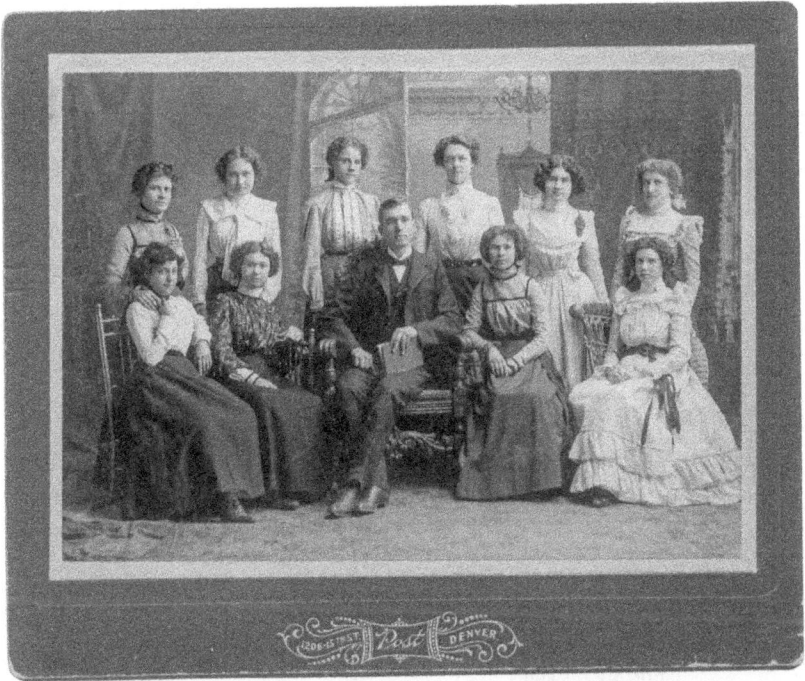

Bruce Leslie and his young ladies' Sunday School class at
People's Tabernacle Congregational Church, Denver, c. 1902

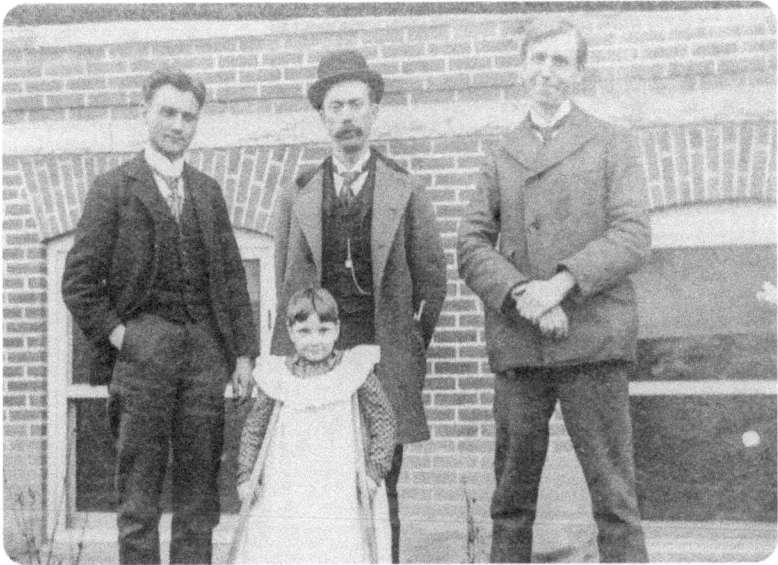

Bruce Leslie, medical student (right), with two classmates
and their successfully treated patient

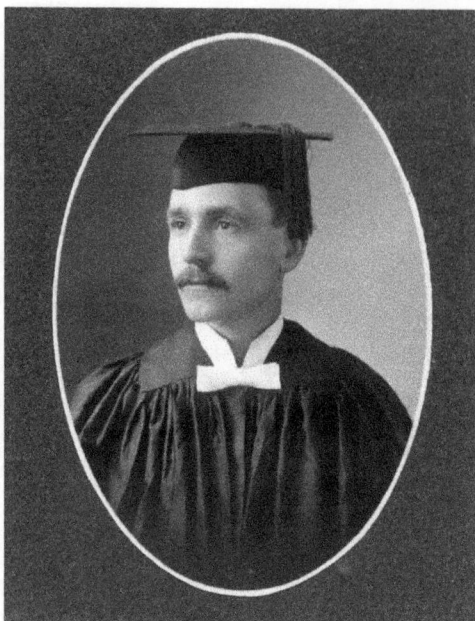

Medical school graduation photograph of Dr. S. B. Leslie
(sporting his short-lived mustache)

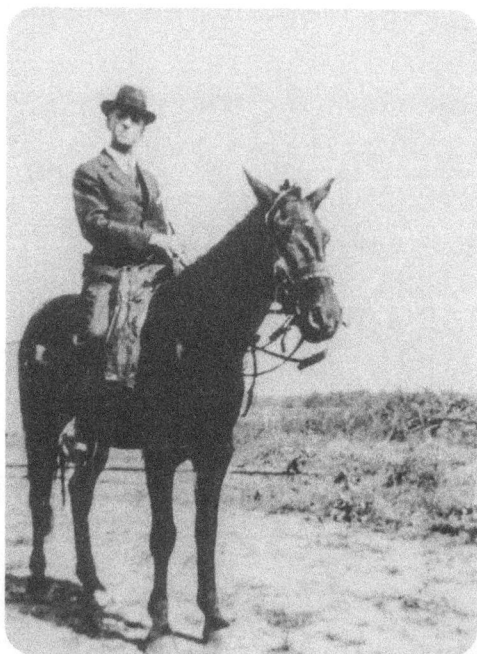

First mode of transportation as a new doctor in Okmulgee, Indian
Territory (before long, the horse would be hitched to his buggy)

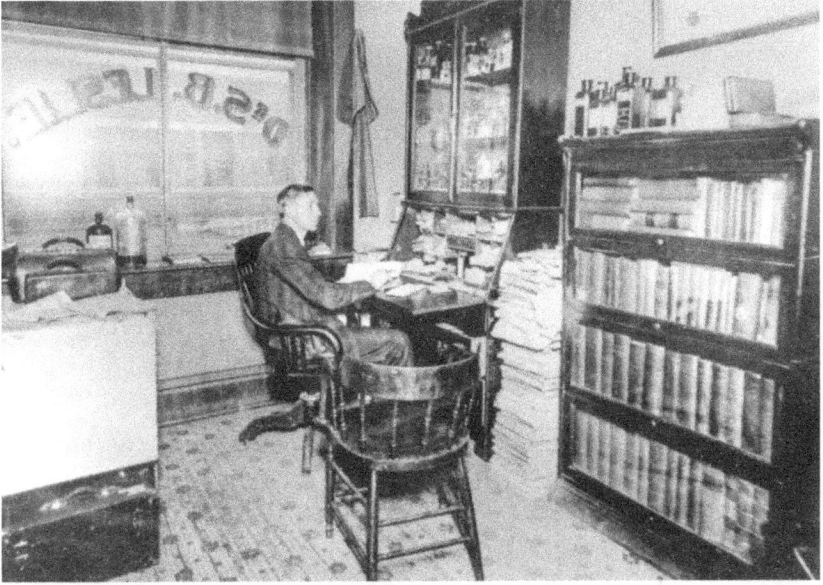

The young doctor in his new office

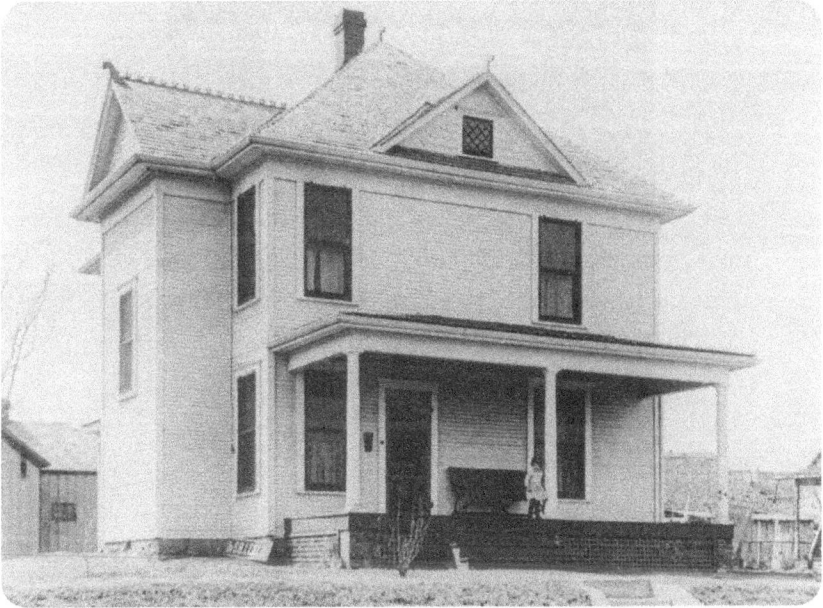

The homestead S. B. Leslie built; c. 1912

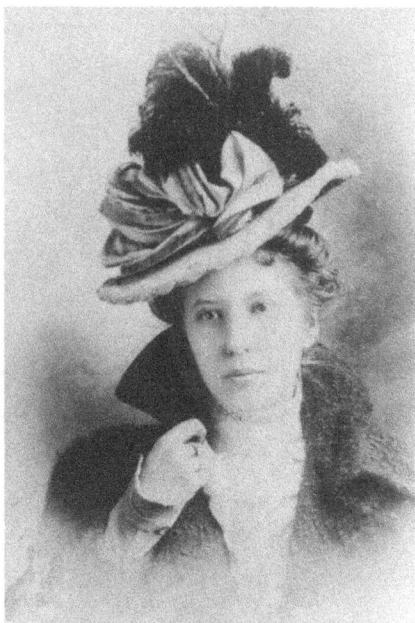

Blossom Eliza McKeage Leslie

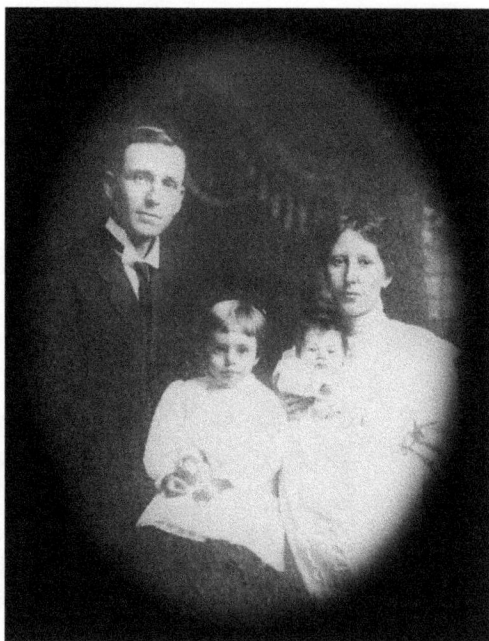

Dr. and Mrs. S. B. Leslie with their eldest daughter,
Elizabeth, and baby, Frances

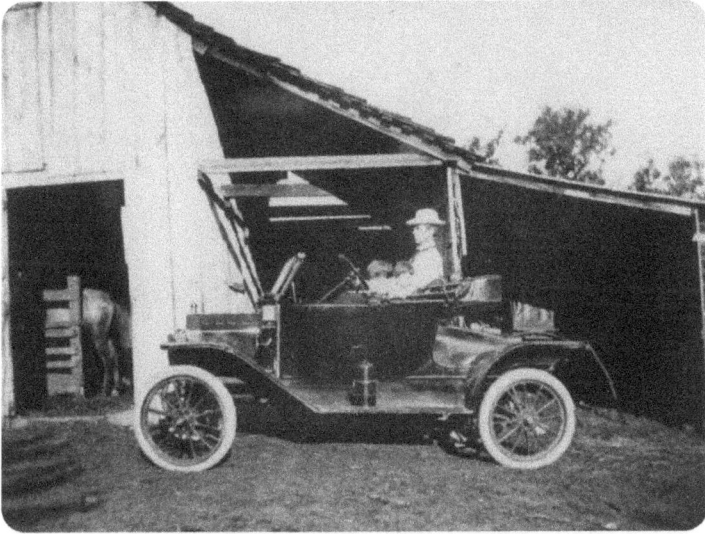

The family's first automobile, a Model T Ford; Elizabeth and
Frances are seated on their father's lap behind the wheel;
note horse in the barn (what must he be thinking?)

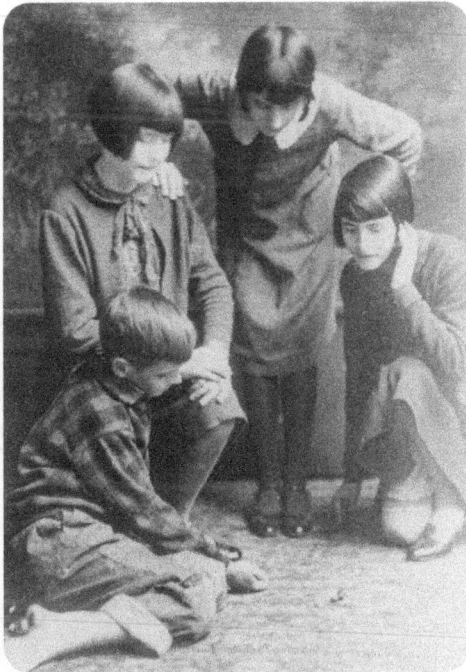

The four Leslie children: clockwise from Sam on the
floor to Frances, Ruth, and Elizabeth

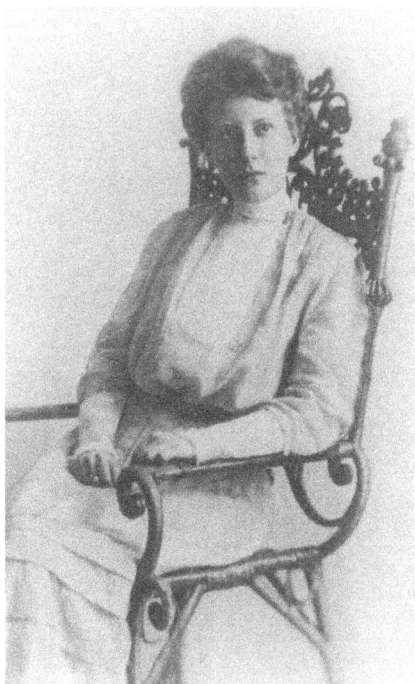

Blossom Leslie

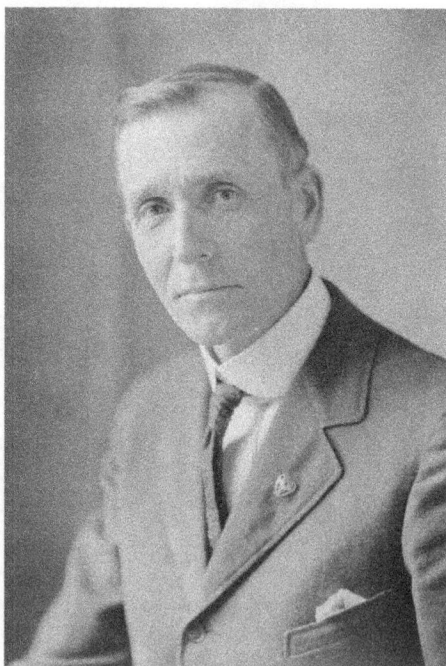

Dr. S. B. Leslie in the 1930s

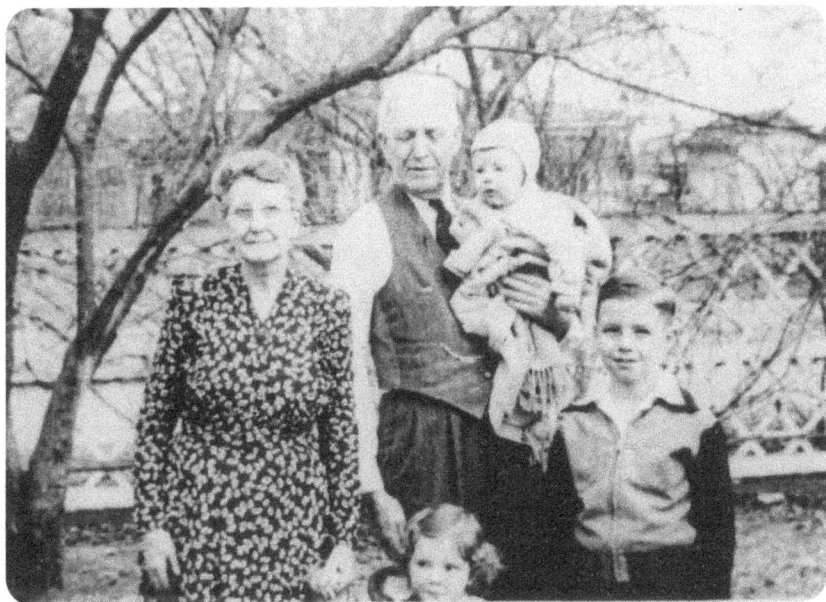

Dr. and Mrs. Leslie with three of their grandchildren; Sam Echols
(in grandfather's arms), Sally Shields (at bottom), and Bruce Shields

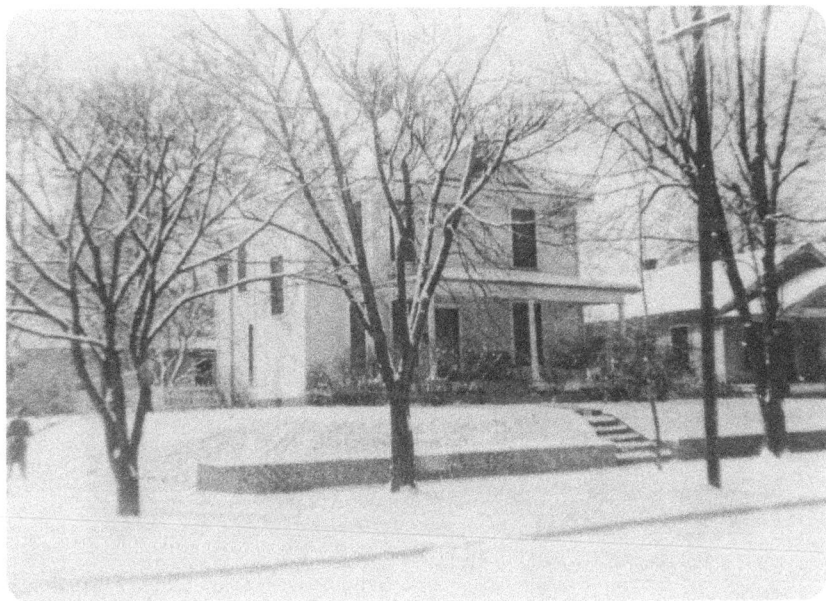

The Leslie homestead around the 1950s, as the grandchildren remember it

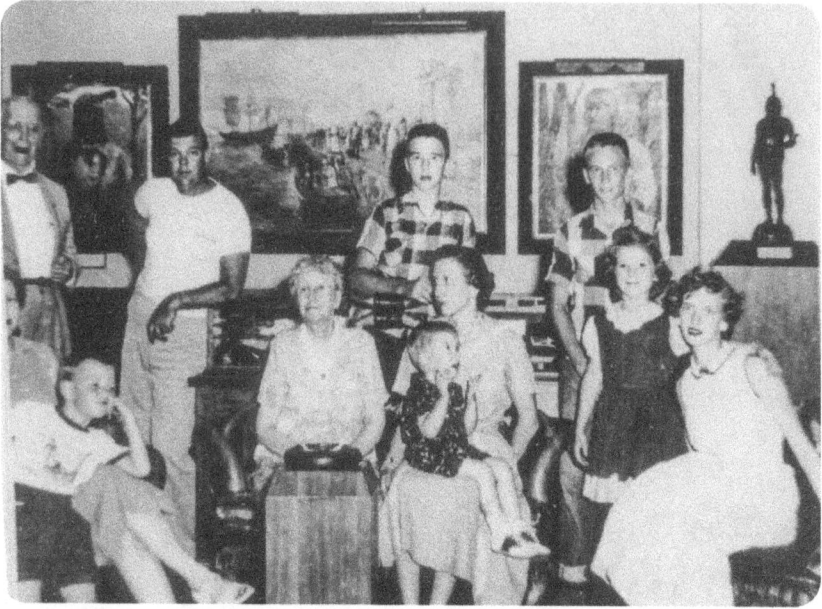

Family at Woolaroc Museum in Bartlesville, Oklahoma, in 1954; standing in back row from left, S. B., Glen Echols, Bruce Shields, and Hal Hunsaker; in front row from left, Frances and Sam Echols, Blossom, Ruth and Chuck Shields, Sally Shields, and Francie Hunsaker

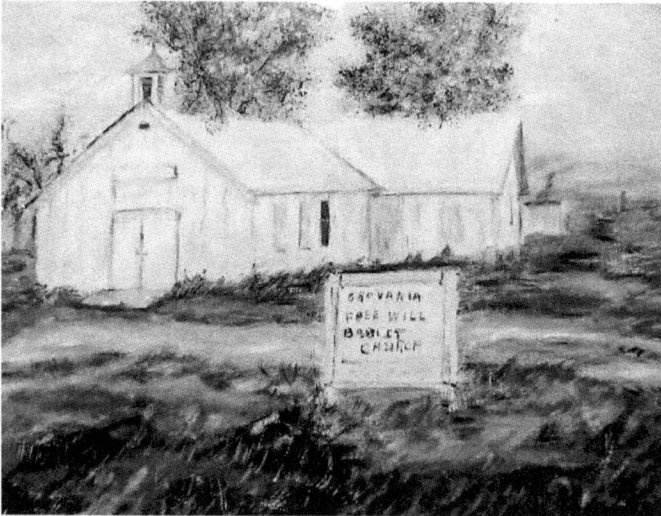

Painting of the original Grovania (artist unknown) that hangs in the new Grovania Free Will Baptist Church

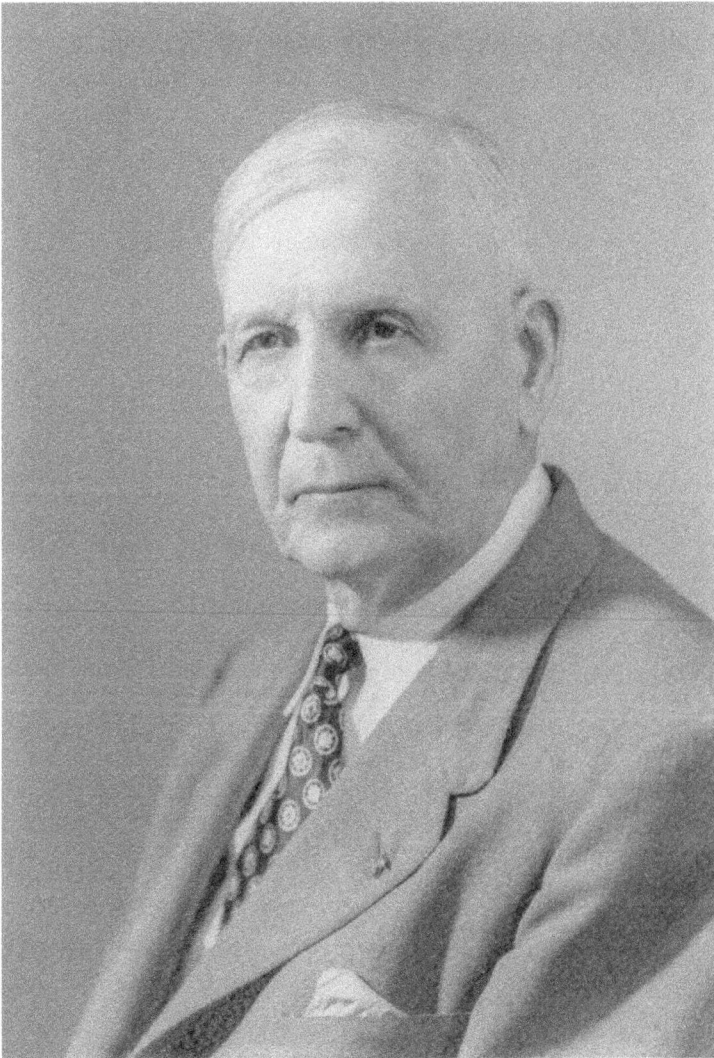

Dr. Samuel Brewster Leslie, Sr.
Last Portrait

PART TWO

Family and Faith

CHAPTER 8

Blossom

I T WAS WELL INTO APRIL, but there was still a dusting of snow on the ground as Blossom Eliza McKeage stepped out through the front door of the Leadville Telephone Company into the late afternoon chill. This was seasonal weather for an altitude of over 10,000 feet, and Blossom paused for a moment to breathe in the crisp, clean air and look up at the snow-capped mountains that surrounded her hometown. She had been fourteen years old when her family moved to Leadville, Colorado, situated in a valley of the Rocky Mountains. That was twelve years ago, and although the harsh climate at first did not agree with her, she had eventually come to love this beautiful part of the world.

Her grandfather, Sumner Coleman, had inherited his father's fortune from real estate and taverns in Chester, Vermont, and had moved west in quest of better weather. He settled near Elgin, Illinois, where he became a gentleman farmer and raised his family. It was there that Blossom's mother, Nettie Coleman, met and married John McKeage, and where Blossom was born on July 23, 1882, in nearby Geneva. She had little memory of Illinois, since her family moved within a few years to Hooper, Nebraska. There she developed many lasting memories, both good and bad: such as the blizzard of 1886, in which some children froze trying to get home; entering school at age five in that intimidating two-story red brick building; her first and only birthday party as a child, when she was seven years old; and those wonderful picnics on the Fourth of July.

As she stepped down the stairs of the telephone company building and walked along the sidewalk, which was lined by Victorian homes, her mind drifted back to those childhood days. It had not been easy for her to leave Hooper. Saying goodbye to her friends and all the happiness she had ever known was hard enough. But the harsh weather of Leadville had added further to her melancholy. And then there were the soldiers. A strike was in progress at the Colorado mines when the McKeages arrived in Leadville, and they had no sooner moved into their new home than the state militia came to town to maintain order and set up camp right beside their house, which Blossom found very unnerving.

Leadville was still a relatively new town when Blossom and her family arrived. It had grown up with the prospectors who came there to mine gold and silver in the 1860s and 70s. Many of the surrounding communities eventually became ghost towns as the mining dried up, but Leadville was more stable because of the railroad, where her father worked. And so her new hometown eventually proved to be a more than suitable place for a teenage girl to grow up.

Rounding the corner toward home, Blossom passed the large, lovely Boehmer home, where her friend, Helen, had once lived. The two girls had quickly become good friends, and Blossom enjoyed many wonderful times in their home. Her thoughts went back to a dinner party, in which it was customary for some of the guests to perform. She had recited a poem called "The Raggedy Man," which she felt went well, thanks to her years of studying elocution. On another occasion, the Boehmers gave a costume party, and Blossom had gone as a colonial lady in a pale yellow dress with a wool-trimmed evening cape. But, of all her memories in that house, the best may have been a grand party in her eighteenth year when she wore her first long dress. It was also a time when she was becoming increasingly noticed by young men, and she had difficulty that evening dividing her attention between two ardent suitors.

Looking back on those school years with Helen and her other friends, she marveled at how the time had flown by. She had enjoyed high school, especially English, Latin, chemistry, and biology, and would have liked to go on with higher learning, but that wasn't to be for most young women in those days. Instead, she would continue her education with a lifetime of reading and other ways of improving her mind. After graduating from high school, she had settled for a job in a local millinery shop. Many of her friends were getting married, and Blossom had several gentleman friends, but was content for the time to live with her parents and her two brothers, Rob and Charlie. She was a year older than Rob and eight years older than Charlie, and both boys adored their sister. They knew she didn't like the name Blossom and eventually took to calling her "Sally," which she liked much better. There had been a third brother, Jay, who died at the age of three, nearly breaking Blossom's heart. For the remainder of her life, it was hard for her to talk about Jay without tears welling up in her eyes.

Blossom had continued working in the millinery shop until she was 21. She was beginning to wonder where her life was heading, when she received an invitation from her grandmother to visit the Coleman farm near Elgin. She accepted and spent seven of the happiest months of her life there. When she returned home, just before Christmas and the New Year of 1905, she took a job with the Leadville Telephone Company, first as a telephone operator and then in the main office. During the next three years, she continued to date several young men and even developed a serious relationship with a fellow named Sid Ganovitz. But something didn't seem right to her, and she eventually suggested to Sid that he should find someone else. So now, as she walked up the steps of her home on that April evening, at the rather advanced age of twenty-six, she could not help but wonder if she would ever meet the right young man. She had prayed about it many times—and she was about to learn that prayers can be answered.

As she entered the house, Blossom was a bit surprised to find the whole family in the living room. She had the feeling that she was the focus of their attention, and yet they all seemed to be studiously avoiding her. The mystery intensified when she noticed that her two brothers were sharing furtive glances and trying to suppress their mirth.

Charlie finally broke the silence by asking, "Can I tell her, Mom?"

"Tell me what?" Blossom asked, now becoming a bit perplexed by all the intrigue.

Her mother smiled with a slight nod toward Charlie, as though to say "Okay."

"You got a letter!" he exclaimed with a huge grin.

"Oh?"

"Yeah! It's from your doctor friend."

My "doctor friend?" The only doctors she knew of in Leadville were older men, and none of them would have any reason to be writing her.

Rob broke in with the explanation. "That one in Oklahoma."

The puzzle suddenly began coming together for Blossom with a shock. Could it possibly be? Her thoughts went back to a summer that now seemed so long ago—the summer of 1900—the summer she had spent in Denver with her cousin Lula Mook—the summer she had met a special young man. He had been a medical student then and the teacher of a young ladies' Sunday School class that she had attended. She almost blushed to remember their times together, especially that last evening at the Mooks' party before she returned to Leadville. He had written her a few times, but then the letters stopped coming, and she had not heard from him in years. She supposed he had found someone else, and that that was the end of it. But she had never forgotten him. She often wondered if her difficulty in accepting the advances of her suitors was that she always held them up to the standard of her young doctor—or at least how she remembered him. Although she did not expect to ever see him again, she had prayed that someday she might find someone just like him.

"Well, are you going to give it to me?" she asked with a smile.

Her father, with a sheepish grin, brought it from behind his back and handed it to her. Sure enough, the return address was Dr. S. B. Leslie of Okmulgee, Oklahoma. She stared at the envelope for a long moment and shook her head in disbelief. Finally, she told her family that she would take it up to her room to read. This seemed to disappoint them, since they were all anxious to know the content of the letter, but each went back to whatever it was they had been pretending to do when she had first come in.

Blossom was surprised to find that her hands were trembling a bit as she held the envelope. She was almost afraid to open it, for fear that the letter would not contain what she hoped to read. But she took a deep breath, said a little prayer, carefully opened the envelope with a pair of scissors, and began to read:

> *Dear Miss McKeage,*
>
> *A great deal of time has passed since we last corresponded, and I trust it has been good to you. I suppose you may be married by now with a family. If not, however, I wonder if I might come to visit. I am planning a trip to Denver this spring and would like to include Leadville in my travels. Please inform me if this would be acceptable.*
>
> *I look forward to your response.*
>
> *Sincerely,*
>
> *S. Brewster Leslie*

She could not suppress a smile as she remembered how proper he always was. But such a brief and cryptic letter! She read it several times, wondering what could be discovered between the lines. But the fact was that he wanted to come for a visit, presumably to see her, and that caused her heart to beat a bit faster, and that caused her to blush.

At dinner that evening, it was unusually silent around the table. Everyone knew what was on one another's mind, especially Blossom. When she could stand it no longer, she finally broke the silence.

"He's coming for a visit," she quietly announced, which prompted smiles and sighs of relief from all her family.

"You gonna marry him, Sally?" Charlie blurted out.

"Of course not, Charlie. I hardly know him."

"But you do like him, don't you?" Rob interjected and glanced over at Charlie with a sly smile that caused both the boys to laugh.

Blossom was now blushing uncontrollably, and her father came to her rescue by changing the topic of conversation.

That evening, Blossom sat at the desk in her room wondering how to compose her response. She decided it should be brief and formal in keeping with the tone of his letter. She went through several sheets of paper, trying to find the right words, and finally settled on a draft that she hoped would be appropriate.

> *Dear Doctor Leslie,*
>
> *Your letter was received with surprise and much pleasure. To answer your question, I have not married. My family and I would be most pleased to have you come to Leadville for a visit during your trip to Denver. We will await the particulars of your itinerary.*
>
> *Sincerely,*
>
> *Blossom McKeage*

She had difficulty falling asleep that night. She kept going over his letter in her mind—the letter that had so suddenly turned her life upside down. And she kept wondering if her response was appropriate. Was it too brief? Should she have been more encouraging? She didn't want to sound too eager, for fear that she might be misinterpreting the intent of his letter. But at the same time she did want him to know that he was more than welcome. Most of all, as she lay in her bed, she thought back to that summer of 1900 and especially to their last time with each other. She remembered how she had felt that evening, knowing they were about to part and that they might never see each other again. She had prayed then that his feelings might be the same as hers. And, just before drifting off to sleep, she said the prayer again.

❦

Bruce Leslie looked out the window of the train as it headed from Denver to Leadville, rumbling along mountainsides and through gorges. He had never been this far west of Denver and marveled at the austere beauty of the land. But his mind was preoccupied with many concerns. For one thing, he had come to realize that he had made a serious miscalculation in planning his trip. Since the Mook family had been so nice to him during his years in Denver, he thought it would be appropriate to pay them a brief visit during his layover in the city. He recognized his mistake when he received a long, effusive response from Lula's mother, Eva Mook, expressing how thrilled the family was to have him come to visit them. She made it a special point to emphasize that her daughter was still single and how wonderful it would be for the two young people to be reunited. He cringed when he read that they were planning a gala party in his honor. That was the absolute last thing he wanted. But, what troubled him most was the realization that Lula and her mother had misinterpreted his intentions. He liked them both, and the last thing he wanted to do was to hurt either one of them—and yet he feared that was exactly what he had just done.

The party had been everything he had dreaded. It seemed that everyone who was anyone in town had been invited. And then there was Lula, looking as lovely as ever in her frilly dress. She had been by his side the entire evening, introducing him to all the guests as though they were already engaged. The party extended into the wee hours, and Bruce finally had to excuse himself, explaining that he had an early morning train to catch. Lula was puzzled when he told her he was going to Leadville, but he didn't provide any explanation, and she was left to wonder what the future held for them.

The other concern that troubled Bruce, as the train continued to rumble through the Rocky Mountains, was whether he was doing the right thing in coming all this way to see someone he had known for only one short summer. What if they discovered, after the passage of time, that they weren't really suited for each other? Would he wound yet another heart? Or would she wound his? He could barely remember what she looked like. The memory he had carried all those years had more to do with her character and her Christian values and the belief that the two of them could raise their children accordingly. Reminding himself of that helped to ease his concerns. And, as the train pulled in to the Leadville station, he looked out the window and saw a beautiful young woman in a simple brown suit, standing on the platform beside her family, and something told him that he had indeed made the right decision.

They took him in their buggy to a hotel in downtown Leadville, where Bruce had made prior arrangements for his lodging. He and Blossom sat side by side, but spoke very little to each other, as they were both rather shy. Most of the conversation came from the two brothers, who pelted Bruce with all sorts of questions about Oklahoma. What were the Indians like? Did they have cowboys? Was it dangerous there? Bruce did his best to answer all their questions in his good-natured way and with his sense of humor, which helped to break the ice.

After he checked in and left his bag in the hotel room, they all continued on to the McKeage home, where he had been invited for dinner. Unlike the ostentatious Mook home, where he had spent the previous evening, Bruce was pleased to see that the McKeage home was modest and cozy, showing good taste and immaculate care. He was also pleased to find how comfortable he was with the entire family. He liked Blossom's parents very much and immediately hit it off with the two boys. At dinner that evening, the conversation flowed pleasantly, with Rob and Charlie again asking most of the questions, and their parents also entering in, while Bruce continued to do his best to keep up. Blossom was the quietest one at the table, which was not unusual for her, but Bruce noticed how she listened to everyone with sincere interest and how her few comments were always articulate and appropriate. As the evening progressed, the two young people found themselves quietly focusing more and more on each other, until it seemed that they were the only ones in the room.

The following day dawned clear and beautiful, with a blue sky that framed the white-capped mountains and a warm sunshine that eased the chill of the mountain air. John McKeage had loaned his smaller buggy to Bruce and Blossom, and they had decided to spend the day at Turquoise Lake, about four and a half miles west of Leadville. As they went slowly down Turquoise Lake Road, both remained rather quiet. They each felt comfortable in the relative silence of the other's company, and yet both could not help wondering what the person beside them might be thinking.

When they arrived at the lake, Bruce could see how it got its name. Although he learned that turquoise had once been mined in the area, he was impressed by how the calm water reflected the turquoise-blue of the sky as well as the aspens and evergreens that rimmed the shoreline. They found a grassy spot near a bank that was bathed in sunlight and laid out a blanket on which they placed the picnic basket that Blossom's mother had prepared. Bruce had many questions that he wanted to ask Blossom about her life and her hopes for the future. And, as they sat in the quiet, tranquil beauty of the moment, he decided that now was the time to begin.

"So, Blossom, tell me about yourself," he began and then immediately chastised himself for such a lame opening.

She had no idea where to begin with such a question. "What do you want to know?" she finally asked.

"Well, what did you enjoy most during your school days?"

"I loved baseball," she offered, after a moment of serious thought.

That was the last thing he expected to hear her say, and he could not suppress a laugh as he tried to picture the demure young lady beside him swinging a bat.

"I'll have you know, sir," she responded with feigned indignation, "that I could run like the wind to make the bases."

"I have no doubt," he retorted, as they shared a good-natured laugh. Then there was another long silence, as Bruce wondered where to take the conversation from there.

"And what did you do when you weren't playing baseball?" he finally queried.

"Well, I was pretty good in school," she admitted with a smile, not adding the fact that she was always at the top of her class. She thought for a moment, remembering a humorous time in her chemistry lab. "The cork got caught in my test tube, so I pulled a hair pin from the back of my hair and used it for a pincher. I didn't know why it made everyone laugh, since it seemed to me like a very logical thing to do."

This got a big laugh out of Bruce, who was learning that his beautiful, intelligent companion also had a charmingly witty side. And so the day went, as they continued to share the stories of their life with each other—both the humorous and the serious. She told him about her time on the Coleman farm and working at the telephone company, and he told her of his experiences as a small town doctor and what it was like living in Oklahoma. As midday eased in to late afternoon, and the trees began casting long shadows across the lake, the topics of their conversation changed from the past to the future. They were both amazed and pleased to learn that they shared the same values and the same hopes and dreams, and that their Christian faith guided it all.

Finally, it came time to head back into Leadville. Again, they enjoyed long spans of silence, but now they both had much to think about. In their brief time together at the lake, it seemed that they had come to know each other in ways that even years of acquaintance often fail to achieve. Each could still not help wondering what the other was thinking—and yet, somehow, they now thought they knew.

The next day was Sunday, and Bruce joined the McKeage family for worship at their Episcopal church. Blossom's mother had a lovely singing voice, a gift she seemed to have inherited from her father, and she sang in their church choir. That morning, she sang the solo part in one of the hymns, which greatly impressed Bruce, much to Blossom's pleasure. If there was ever a single moment that sealed the fate of the two young people, it may well have been that morning, sitting side by side in church singing together, listening intently to the sermon together, praying together. Before the service was over, Bruce knew beyond a doubt that this was the woman he wanted by his side in worship and in life for the rest of his days. And the woman by his side felt the same.

That afternoon, the whole family took a trip to Twin Lakes, a town near Leadville that had enjoyed a transient mining boom and had remained a popular tourist destination since the late 1870s. Again, Bruce found himself on the bank of a lake of breathtaking beauty. But at that moment he had something else on his mind. After the family had finished their picnic lunch, he asked Blossom if they might go for a walk along the lakefront. And, as the rest of the family sat, wondering what might be coming next, the two young folks wandered off together.

The night before, Bruce had had a serious talk with Mr. McKeage about his aspirations for the future and ended by asking permission to propose to his daughter. This was what the father was hoping to hear, and, after giving his enthusiastic blessing, he could not wait to tell his wife. So, as her family remained on their picnic blanket that Sunday afternoon, Blossom's parents were fairly confident about what their daughter and her suitor were likely to be discussing, while Rob and Charlie could make a pretty good guess.

The two were gone for what seemed to the family like a rather long time, while the four of them sat in anxious silence. By the time they finally saw them coming back around the bend in the lake, their curiosity had reached a fevered pitch, and they all stood up with big grins on their faces, preparing to receive some special news. But Blossom and Bruce were frustratingly silent. They smiled casually and allowed that they had a pleasant walk, but offered nothing more. Everyone wanted to ask, but no one dared. Even Charlie was able to restrain himself. Had Bruce changed his mind? Or lost his nerve? Had Blossom refused? Had they even discussed marriage? And so they quietly picked up their blanket and basket and headed home.

That evening, around a simple meal of soup and bread, the tension in the dining room was palpable. The awkward silence was only intermittently broken by someone's attempt to make conversation. "It was a nice day." "Yes, a nice day." And everyone would nod their head in agreement and then fall back into silence. They avoided eye contact, except for an occasional furtive glance right or left, knowing what was on everyone's mind. Finally, Blossom felt that she could hold back no longer.

"Bruce and I have an announcement to make," she said in a barely audible voice.

Suddenly, the silence was even deeper, as her family all leaned forward with their eyes riveted on Blossom. But she simply smiled and turned her head to look into Bruce's eyes, as though to say, "Your turn."

Bruce swallowed and tried to look appropriately serious, as he proceeded to make the announcement.

"This afternoon at the lake, with Mr. McKeage's permission, I asked Blossom if she would be my wife."

Blossom blushed, and all her family sucked in a deep breath as though they were surprised to hear exactly what they had been hoping to hear. But Bruce seemed to have said all he intended to say, and the silence resumed. It was Charlie who broke it by blurting out what all of them were thinking.

"Did ya say yes, Sally!!"

To which Blossom, with a growing smile, quietly nodded in the affirmative. Then the celebration exploded, as the boys jumped up, shouting. Mr. McKeage walked around the table to shake Bruce's hand, and Mrs. McKeage, with a tear in her eye, hugged her daughter.

Bruce was scheduled to return home the following morning, and the entire McKeage family went with him to the Leadville station. The night before, following the big announcement, they had all sat together in the living room and talked about the future. After they were married, Blossom explained, she would be moving to Okmulgee, where Bruce had a thriving practice and had recently built a large home. However, the young couple had agreed that propriety dictated a respectable length of time be allowed for their engagement, and it would be the better part of a year before Bruce would return to Leadville for the wedding.

As they stood on the station platform, the little group was rife with conflicting emotions. Blossom's family was overjoyed for her but were already thinking about how much they were going to miss her. Blossom too was struggling with her emotions, as she considered her good fortune, but felt the pain of saying goodbye, for what seemed like such a long time, to the man she had just come to love. Only Bruce seemed to be in control of his emotions, at least on the surface, as he shook hands with each of Blossom's family and then turned to face her. Although they could not bring themselves to kiss in public, the look in their eyes said it all. And, as Bruce mounted the steps of the train, he felt a lump in his throat and a gentle breeze swirling about his head.

❧

In the months that followed, time seemed to move slowly for the young couple, although both had much to occupy their days. Bruce had to work extra hard when he got back to make up for the time he had been away from his patients, and the demand for his attention never seemed to let up. Blossom continued to work at the telephone company and filled much of her free time planning and preparing for the wedding. And both of them paused many times each day to thank God for their blessings.

They had agreed to write often, and both proved true to their promise. With time, their letters became longer and somewhat more familiar, although they both retained a certain formality in their writing style, a trait that would characterize Bruce's correspondence throughout his life. One of the issues that continued to bother him was his last encounter with Lula Mook and her mother, and he shared his concern with Blossom in one of his letters:

June 9, 1908

Dear Blossom,

> *Your last letter was a source of much pleasure. No doubt Mrs. Mook was (and is yet) quite jealous of you for Lula. She felt for some reason that I had made the trip to Colorado for a companion. And she inadvertently asked me about you. I think she could not convince herself I was not corresponding with you.*

> *Mrs. Mook is over anxious for her daughter. I have a great deal I might tell you when I see you Blossom.*

He then went into a lengthy description of the American Indians around Okmulgee, in response to some concerns that Blossom had expressed, and ended the letter:

> *For fear I will tire you of this subject I will close with best wishes to you My dear friend.*

> *S. Brewster Leslie*

And so it went through the remainder of 1908 and into the spring of 1909. In June of that year, Bruce returned to Leadville for their long-awaited wedding on the sixteenth day of the month. His only disappointment was that his mother had decided it was too far and expensive for her and her daughters to travel. She said they would be preparing their home for the newlyweds and she would meet her new daughter-in-law then. So the only family at the wedding on the

Leslie side were his two cousins, who were still living in Denver. But, of course, all of Blossom's family and many of their friends in town were in attendance and filled the McKeage home, where they were married.

Their wedding day dawned cool and clear. Blossom wore a blue wool suit with a matching hat and carried a bouquet of real orange blossoms. The only detraction from an otherwise perfect day was when her emotions so overwhelmed her that her face broke out in a rash. But a little makeup can do wonders, and Bruce thought he had never seen her look more radiant. In his eyes, she was the most beautiful woman in the world—the woman with whom he would spend the remainder of his days. And, when Blossom looked at her handsome doctor in his new suit, she could only marvel at her good fortune. As they stood together in front of family, friends, and God, their two hearts swelled with pride and thanksgiving when the preacher pronounced them "man and wife."

During their long-distance correspondences, they had shared thoughts about where to spend their honeymoon. Bruce raised the possibility of going to Arkansas, so that Blossom could meet some of his family. He would be proud to show her his birthplace, Leslie, the town named after his grandfather, which was currently enjoying a boom of prosperity. And he would also take great pride in showing off his beautiful bride to the folks back home.

Visiting relatives was probably not Blossom's first choice for their honeymoon, although she did welcome the opportunity to meet her new in-laws. And she very much wanted to do whatever would make her husband happy. Furthermore, Bruce had sweetened the deal by adding that they would stop along the way at a popular resort community, which would be a most appropriate honeymoon destination—a place called Eureka Springs.

In the northwest corner of Arkansas, some eighty miles from the town of Leslie, there is a cluster of crystal clear springs, whose curative waters were known to the indigenous people long before the arrival of the white man. In the 1850s, a pioneer doctor by the name of Alvah Jackson discovered that the spring water cured his son's eye injury. This led him to market "Dr. Jackson's Eye-Water," launching the reputation of the region that became known as "Indian Healing Spring," with sparkling spring waters that purportedly could cure almost anything. After the Civil War, it became a popular health resort and eventually a thriving community with many luxurious Victorian homes, and in 1879, the town was renamed Eureka Springs.

The flagship of the town was the Crescent Hotel, which opened in 1886 and soon became known as "The Grand Old Lady of the Ozarks." Positioned on a high ridge overlooking the town, the hotel was a wonder of its day. Constructed of limestone from a nearby quarry, it rose five stories and was topped by three turret-shaped roofs. It had 100 large rooms with high ceilings, wide corridors, and lovely verandas, all exquisitely furnished and lighted by Edison lamps. The spacious, manicured gardens that surrounded the hotel, with their Victorian gazebos and the Wedding Court, added the ideal finishing touch to an attraction that, by the turn of the century, had become a popular destination for travelers from far and wide. And among those visitors, on the afternoon of June 18, 1909, was a young couple who signed in at the registration desk of the hotel as Dr. and Mrs. S. B. Leslie.

They had left Leadville early on the morning after their wedding day and were accompanied to the train station by Blossom's entire family. A few of their friends were also there to see them off, and they tossed flowers as the newlyweds made their way across the platform amid laughter and shouts of best wishes. The young couple waved as they boarded the train and again as they took their seats and looked out the window. Blossom had a tear in her eye as she saw her parents and brothers standing on the platform and wondered when she would see them again. But, as the train pulled out, she looked over at her handsome husband sitting beside her and could only think how blessed she was.

The day was bright and warm, and by early afternoon they had passed through Denver and were leaving the mountains far behind. Ahead of them lay grassy prairies and then the farmlands of Kansas. Blossom had never seen such flat land, with hardly a tree in sight, and it seemed to add to her growing feeling of homesickness. Bruce sensed her emotions and tried to comfort her by recalling how he had also felt the first time he saw such wide-open land. He assured her that where they were going in Arkansas and Oklahoma would be more like what she had known back home. Blossom may not have been convinced, but she appreciated her husband's attempt to cheer her up.

It was dark by the time they pulled into the Kansas City station, where they were scheduled to change trains. The layover barely gave them enough time to find a quick bite to eat, and then they were off again on the next leg of their journey. As the train rumbled through the darkness, the young couple tried to get some sleep, and it seemed that they had just drifted off when morning sunshine came through their window. As they continued south through Missouri, Blossom noticed that the terrain was changing, just as Bruce had promised. The flat land was giving way to hills of increasing size that were densely covered in verdant woodlands. It wasn't the majestic mountains she had known in Colorado, but it somehow made her feel that she could breath more freely. By early afternoon, they had crossed into Arkansas, and soon the train was pulling into the Eureka Springs station.

They took a hotel carriage up a winding road to the Crescent Hotel. Despite their fatigue from the long trip, they were far too excited to think about taking a nap. The grandeur of the hotel, its magnificent surroundings, and the breathtaking vista across the valley below captivated them, and they spent the rest of the afternoon walking around the hotel gardens and relaxing in rocking chairs on the veranda. That evening, in the stately dining room, they enjoyed their first real meal together as husband and wife. The next day, after a relaxed, hearty breakfast, they went back downtown to explore the quaint shops and sip the cold water that came from the many springs in the area. It was a magical experience for Blossom— her honeymoon—which she would savor for the rest of her life. That evening, they turned in early, because they had a train to catch at the crack of dawn.

They rushed through a light breakfast, checked out of the hotel, and returned to the Eureka Springs station for the train to Leslie, eighty miles away. The train wound slowly through the Ozark hills and mountains, and it was approaching noon by the time they pulled into the recently built Leslie station. As Blossom looked out the window of their coach, she was surprised to see a large number of people waving at them from the station platform, and soon learned that most were members of the Leslie family. She could not recall ever seeing Bruce so excited, and she vowed to suppress her shyness and do her best to fit in.

Bruce was indeed thrilled to be back with his family after so many years and to present his new wife to them. It seemed that nearly every Leslie who still lived in the area had come to greet them, and they all crowded around Bruce, shaking his hand, patting him on the back and hugging him, while Blossom stood quietly to the side. She was beginning to wonder if anyone cared about her, when Bruce recognized his omission and rushed over to begin the long series of introductions, as she smiled, extended her hand, and blushed.

They all went to Andrew's large home on the corner of the two main streets in downtown Leslie, where they spent the afternoon talking—the men in one room and the women in another. Bruce especially enjoyed talking with his Uncle John, since the two doctors had much to share about the evolving state of medicine. Blossom enjoyed talking with the women, and before long was beginning to feel comfortable as a new member of the Leslie family. However, she also found it tiring to be the constant focus of attention and was not sorry when it was time to leave Leslie and begin the final leg of their journey to Okmulgee.

Dusk was beginning to settle over the town as the train pulled in to the Okmulgee station. The exhausted couple looked out the window in search of familiar faces, but saw none. Bruce was not surprised that no one in his family had come to greet them, since his mother had made it rather clear that they would meet his new wife when the newlyweds arrived at the house. Accordingly, Bruce had made arrangements for a buggy and driver to meet them at the station and take them to their home.

It was dark by the time they reached the house, and Blossom felt a twinge of apprehension as she looked up at the imposing white structure on the hill with dim lights coming from some of the windows. She found it hard to imagine that this was where she would spend the remainder of her life and where she would be the "lady of the house." Bruce carried their bags up the concrete stairs from the street to the porch at the back of the house. It was quiet inside, and Bruce knocked on the door, hoping not to alarm anyone. Ollie opened the door, and when she saw her step-brother, she gave out a loud squeal of delight that brought her sister and mother into the room. They all hugged Bruce and fussed over him, while Blossom again stood quietly in the shadows, waiting her turn. When the sisters finally seemed to notice her, they looked to Bruce for an introduction.

"I would like all of you to meet Blossom McKeage—I mean Blossom Leslie," he quickly corrected himself with an embarrassed grin that made Blossom blush. "She is my wife," he felt it necessary to explain.

"We know that," Ona laughed, and both sisters rushed over to hug their new sister-in-law. But their mother kept her distance, as though she was expecting Blossom to come to her.

"You are welcome in our home, my dear," the mother said, with only the hint of a smile. A moment of awkward silence followed, and then Blossom walked over to acknowledge her new mother-in-law. She wondered if maybe she should curtsy, but then the matriarch offered her hand, which Blossom took for the brief time before it was withdrawn.

"Thank you, Ma'am," was all she could think to say.

"Our home, not your home," Blossom thought, as she lay in her new bed that first night. Her mind was a jumble of emotions. She was lonely. She missed her parents and brothers. She missed Leadville. She missed the mountains. And now she wondered if she was even welcome in her own home. The two sisters had been friendly enough, and she had a feeling that they would all get along well. But she was perplexed by Bruce's mother, who seemed to want her to understand who was the true "lady of the house." As she lay there thinking about it all, she tried to give her mother-in-law the benefit of the doubt. She was obviously very proud of her son and probably felt that no woman was entirely worthy of him. And, after living in the house for nearly two years, she had become accustomed to being in charge, and it was understandable that it would be hard to relinquish that.

And, with those thoughts, Blossom drifted off to sleep on that first night in her new home, but she couldn't help wondering what the future held for her.

The days that followed passed slowly for Blossom. Bruce had gone back to his office the morning after their arrival, leaving her alone with the three women. Life in the household turned out to be much as she had anticipated. Callie Marrs was clearly in charge, and her two daughters took that in stride. With time, Blossom acquiesced to her role as another of Callie's daughters, allowing her mother-in-law to make most of the decisions in their daily lives. Inwardly, she resented it, but she knew that Bruce loved his mother and that he was oblivious to how she dominated their life at home. And so she kept quiet in the interest of their domestic tranquility.

As Blossom had anticipated, she got along very well with Ona and Ollie. The three young women enjoyed cooking and sewing together and working jigsaw puzzles, a pastime that would become one of Blossom's favorites throughout her life. But she missed not being able to spend more time with her husband. It seemed that Bruce was always working. He left early each morning and rarely got home before suppertime. And he went to bed early because he never knew when he would be called out at night. After this had gone on for a month or so, Blossom decided that something had to change. And then one night an opportunity presented itself.

The family was all asleep when the phone rang, and Bruce got up to answer it. When he came back to their bedroom, he whispered to Blossom that he had to go out to see a patient who was about to deliver her baby. This was the opportunity that she had been waiting for, and to his surprise, she announced that she was going with him.

"Are you sure?" he asked, with a note of surprise. "It could be a long night."

"Don't you think I can take it?" she responded with the same feigned indignation that he had first seen at Turquoise Lake. "I might even be able to help you."

He could only smile, as he began to realize what a remarkable woman he had married.

"All right, then. But we must hurry."

Bruce now owned a shiny new buggy, and he quickly hitched his horse to it and helped Blossom up onto the seat beside him. He explained that their destination was a farm a little over a mile outside of town. They were both quiet as they rode along the dirt road. He was most likely thinking about the steps he would need to take when they reached the farmhouse. And she was thinking about how proud she was to be sitting beside the town's leading doctor. And both may have been remembering that first time they rode together in a horse and buggy back in Colorado.

When they arrived at the farmhouse, Blossom proved true to her word that she would be able to help her husband. She boiled water and held the hand of the young mother, giving her moral support, as Bruce skillfully brought another new life into the world. When it was all over, they sat for a while with the happy family, marveling at the miracle of life. Bruce and Blossom looked over at each other and undoubtedly had the same thought in their minds.

It was a cloudless, moonlit summer night, as the doctor and his wife bid the new mother and her family goodbye. The air was warm and sweet with the fragrance of hay in the meadows and the pine trees beside the country road. Blossom noticed that Bruce was driving more slowly than when they had come out to the farm. He seemed to be enjoying the moment. She moved a little closer to him and rested her hand on his. He kept looking straight ahead, but she could see the smile on his face and feel the gentle warmth of his hand against hers. And so the young couple held hands in silence as the buggy continued slowly down the moonlit lane.

CHAPTER 9

Family

I T WAS A COLD FEBRUARY MORNING and still dark outside when the old
alarm clock once again split the stillness of the bedroom. Bruce
reached over to silence it and then sank back into the soft, warm
bed. He had been up twice during the night on house calls and
desperately needed more sleep but knew that was not an option. He
did, however, allow himself a couple of minutes of quiet meditation
and reflection before getting up.

When he had chosen to pursue the practice of medicine, he
was not entirely unaware of how difficult it would be. But it was
only after experiencing it for himself that he fully understood what
a challenging profession he had entered. Not only were the hours
long—he literally had to be available whenever his patients needed
him, twenty-four hours a day, seven days a week—but there was
also the awesome responsibility for the life and well-being of other
people. Some days, especially when he was critically low on sleep,
he questioned whether he was up to the task. But then he would
experience the rewarding feeling of having made life better for one
of his patients, and that seemed to assuage any doubt that this was
how God had intended for him to devote his life.

And so, after a brief prayer of thanksgiving, he quietly slipped out
of bed, trying not to disturb Blossom. Resting his feet on the small
braided rug to avoid the icy hardwood floor, he slowly unfolded the
full length of his lanky six-foot frame and enjoyed a long, luxurious
stretch. Then he slipped on his house shoes and headed softly down

the hall toward their one bathroom, taking special care not to wake the baby.

As he walked by the nursery, Bruce could not resist peeking in at little Elizabeth, who lay snuggled in peaceful sleep. Since her arrival last August, in the year 1910, she had become the center of their world. Neither parent could get over how blessed they felt to have such a beautiful, healthy bundle of joy. But it hadn't all been easy, as they discovered the challenges of young parenthood. For nearly the first six months, Elizabeth had not slept well, and there had been many restless nights, especially for Blossom, who did her best to see that the doctor got as much sleep as possible. For the past month, however, Elizabeth had slept through the night more times than not. And, on that morning, Bruce hoped to keep it that way.

He shaved and combed his hair and quickly ran a warm washrag over his upper body before returning to the bedroom to dress. One thing he never had to worry about was what to wear. It was always the same. Few people ever saw him in anything but a starched, long-sleeve white shirt and dark dress trousers, and that is what he slipped into that morning. Later, he would add a bow tie and dress shoes, but for the moment he relished the freedom and comfort of an open collar and his slippers.

He walked gingerly down the oak stairs to the foyer and then stepped out onto the front porch to retrieve the morning paper. This was his favorite time of day. The sun was just rising, sending the first rays of light into the dawn sky. Bruce looked up in awesome wonder, as he did most every morning, at the vastness and the beauty of God's creation. The quietness and majesty of the moment never failed to give him a sense of closeness with God, and he closed his eyes in silence and allowed a feeling of profound thankfulness to wash over him.

One thing that Blossom had learned early on about her husband was that he was the epitome of frugality. Although he was always generous with his money, never hesitating to help those in need, he could not abide wasting a penny. And so it was that the house was freezing that wintry morning because, with the exception of the nursery, they always turned the heat off at night—that was what blankets were for. His next routine, therefore, was to light the gas stove in the living room, so it would start warming up the house before Blossom came down.

In the kitchen, he started the coffee and then sat down in a straight chair and picked up his Bible. This was another of his most cherished times of the day—the quiet time when he could read a passage of scripture and meditate on its meaning. He had recently started to reread Psalms, and he smiled to realize that today he would be reading the twenty-third chapter—one of his favorites. When he got to the fifth verse—"my cup runneth over"—he paused to think of his young wife and their beautiful baby sleeping soundly upstairs, and he considered once again how truly blessed he was. After finishing the chapter, he closed his eyes for a time of silent prayer. And this was how he continued to begin each day for the remainder of his life.

When the coffee was ready, he poured a cup and sat back down to read the morning paper—the *Okmulgee Democrat*. The headlines, as on most days, described the latest activities of the Taft administration, which had become increasingly troubling to Bruce. He was a staunch Lincoln Republican and had been a loyal supporter of President Roosevelt. When TR had recommended Taft to succeed him, Bruce had enthusiastically voted for him, but now he was having second thoughts. While Roosevelt had advanced a progressive agenda that seemed to favor the welfare of the common people, it appeared more and more that Taft was being swayed toward the interests of corporate America. Roosevelt had also begun to express his concern, and Bruce wondered what TR might do about it.

Just as he was beginning to get a bit worked up about the nation's political affairs, Blossom walked into the kitchen and brought him back to what was really important in his life. She kissed the top of his head, and he put his arm around her slender waist. They cherished these moments alone together, especially since they had not always enjoyed a great deal of privacy in their own home. Ever since Blossom arrived, her mother-in-law, Callie, had continued to be the dominant "woman of the house." Bruce may have never fully recognized the problem, since both women did their best to shelter him from domestic issues so he could concentrate on running his practice and providing for his family. In any case, things changed significantly with the arrival of Elizabeth.

After he had completed construction of the family homestead to which he brought his mother and two step-sisters, Bruce built two smaller houses on his adjacent property, with plans to rent them out for additional income. But, with the impending birth of their first child, it was decided that Callie's room would be needed for the nursery, and that Callie should move into one of the smaller houses next door, which she did with considerable reluctance. Ona had already married and moved across town, and Ollie was now working as the society editor for the local paper. It was felt that Ollie should stay in the main house to help Blossom with the baby—at least that was the plan.

Bruce watched his wife as she prepared their breakfast, and then they sat together at the kitchen table, held hands, and gave thanks. Breakfast was one of the few quiet times they had together in those early days of their married life, although even they were numbered. Already, Blossom had to eat rather quickly so she could go back up to feed Elizabeth and then come back downstairs to prepare breakfast for Ollie, who would be coming downstairs around nine before leaving for the newspaper office. That barely gave Blossom time to clean up the kitchen before starting preparation of their noon meal.

And so it went in those early days. Bruce would leave the house a little before eight and walk the few blocks to his office to begin another long day, while Blossom would begin the seemingly endless tasks of keeping the home fires burning. Whenever he could, Bruce would come home for lunch and then take a brief nap on the living room sofa before going back to his office or to make house calls. Dinnertime depended on when he could get away from the demands of his patients, but Blossom always had it ready whenever he arrived. They went to bed early, since Bruce never knew when he would be called out in the middle of the night, and both of them were usually exhausted from their long day. Before turning in, however, they typically enjoyed a quiet interlude together, when Elizabeth was asleep, and they could sit and read or talk or just enjoy the silence. And yet even that brief respite would soon be a distant memory they would look back on longingly.

Elizabeth's childhood, as with most children, was a mixture of pure joy interspersed with moments of sheer panic. One of the latter occurred during the first spring of her life. Blossom had continued to accompany Bruce on some of his calls into the country and now took Elizabeth with them. The weather was beginning to turn warm, and Blossom bundled their little baby up in a soft blanket and took her seat beside the doctor in the buggy with Elizabeth in her arms. As they were leaving town, they passed an oil-well pump house, and the engine in the building suddenly backfired, spooking their horse and causing it to rear up and throw the buggy out of control. Bruce struggled to hold on to the reins and steady the buggy, and Blossom reached for something to keep from falling out. In the process, she lost her hold on Elizabeth, who went flying out of the buggy to the grass beside the road. Looking back on it, both parents agreed that it was the worst moment of fear and panic either had ever known. As they rushed to where the small bundle lay motionless, they knew she must be dead. But, when they got to her, she looked up at them with nothing more than a puzzled and somewhat frightened expression on her little face. Bruce checked her over carefully and found that she had suffered no injuries. The blanket had apparently protected her, but both parents were convinced that something greater than that had saved the life of their child that evening. And, with tears running down their cheeks, they held hands and shared a deep and sincere prayer of thanks.

As Elizabeth gradually transitioned from infancy to young childhood, her parents marveled at how each day seemed to bring new wonders in her development. But it also brought increasing demands, especially on her mother, to whom Elizabeth had become tenaciously attached. And it was that closeness between mother and daughter that contributed to the next family crisis. Several cases of smallpox were appearing in Okmulgee, to which Bruce had apparently acquired immunity through exposure to so many of his patients. But Blossom had not been so fortunate. She came down with the illness and had to be quarantined to her bedroom. Of course, little Elizabeth could not understand what was happening, and she would come to her mother's door and cry, "Mama, Mama," which almost broke Blossom's heart. Eventually, Elizabeth also contracted a mild form of the disease, but still had to be kept from her mother to avoid making her condition more severe. Bruce, of course, was very knowledgeable and skillful at managing patients with smallpox, and both mother and daughter got by with mild cases. And so another crisis passed, only to be followed by more.

By the time Elizabeth was approaching her second year of life, she had gone from walking to running like the wind, and her mother tried to never let her out of her sight—at least to the extent that was possible. In the barn behind their house, Bruce kept their horse, some chickens, and a cow. One evening, as he was milking the cow and Blossom was momentarily distracted, Elizabeth slipped out of the house and ran to the barn. Her mother came running out to get her, but Elizabeth was in her playful "catch me" mood and, to Blossom's horror, darted under the cow. She was sure the cow was going to kick and kill her daughter, but the little girl just laughed and ran back out from behind the cow. Bruce also laughed, but Blossom saw no humor in the affair whatsoever and let both father and daughter know that she was not at all pleased with either of them.

As the world entered the year 1912, events were unfolding at home and abroad, and also in the Leslie family, that would be remembered with both tears and smiles. In the spring, the world was shocked by news of the RMS *Titanic* sinking on her maiden voyage, with the loss of more than 1,500 lives. Blossom, with her tender heart, cried when she heard the news, and Elizabeth could only wonder what made her mother so sad. That summer, Theodore Roosevelt, having lost the Republican nomination to President Taft, formed the Progressive Party, soon to be known as the Bull Moose Party, which nominated him to take another run at the presidency. And that gave Elizabeth's father a reason to smile. But the greatest joy for the family that year was to come in the fall.

When the year was still young, Blossom had discovered that something was again changing, and before long she informed Bruce that their second child was on the way. In September of that year, she gave birth to a chubby, beautiful little red-haired girl, whom they named Frances Jeanette. Almost from the day she was born, it was clear that Frances would have a very different personality from that of her older sister. As Elizabeth had grown older, she displayed an increasingly serious and responsible demeanor. Frances, on the other hand, seemed to have been born with a twinkle in her eyes and a constant smile on her rosy lips. And, as the two sisters continued to develop, the contrast between their personalities became ever more striking, with Frances as the seemingly carefree, bubbly, irrepressible child, a persona that would largely define her throughout her life.

In the meantime, Bruce's optimism on the national political front turned to dismay when Woodrow Wilson defeated both Roosevelt and Taft for the presidency. He and Blossom could not help but worry about the future of their country with a Democrat back in the White House. But that disappointment paled in comparison to the great sadness that was to shake their family before the year came to an end.

Bruce made a practice of checking in on his mother, in her home beside theirs, each evening when he got home. One night, he entered the house and called her name, but there was no response. He went back to her bedroom and found Callie lying on the bed unable to talk or move one side of her body. He recognized that his mother had suffered a stroke. He checked her vital signs and, once he was sure she was stable, he hurried next door to inform Blossom and Ollie and bring them over to help care for her. After sitting with Callie and comforting her for a long time, the two women changed her into a nightgown and eased her under the covers. One of them stayed with her around the clock, feeding her and doing the best they could to make her comfortable. There was very little more that could be done for a stroke victim in those days. Bruce sat beside his mother as often as he could, and his thoughts must have gone back to a time when he was a young boy and had sat next to his dying father. Ever since moving out of the main house, Callie had seemed increasingly depressed, and now with this latest affliction she showed very little will to live. One evening, with Bruce by her side, she closed her eyes for the last time.

And so, as 1912 came to an end, Bruce and Blossom sat with their little family around the Christmas tree counting their blessings. And they had much to be thankful for. Ona and her husband had come over, and Ollie was there with a serious suitor. Frances lay in her mother's arms, enthralled by the twinkling lights on the tree, while Elizabeth played happily at her mother's feet. But there was also a sadness in the room because of the one person who was absent. Despite their differences, Blossom had wept bitterly at the funeral, and Bruce felt an emptiness in his heart as anyone must when losing their mother.

◌ ∵ ◌

During his first ten years of medical practice in Okmulgee, Bruce Leslie progressed through several different modes of transportation. When he first arrived in his new hometown, his main way of getting around was on his two feet. This had worked reasonably well for making local house calls, since most of the homes were clustered around the downtown area. When he had to call on a family in the country, he would rent a horse from the livery stable. As his practice grew, however, renting became increasingly impractical and, as soon as he was able, he purchased his own horse—his second mode of transportation. It was a fine chestnut horse on which the doctor looked very distinguished as he rode out of town wearing his suit and tie and a stylish fedora. Riding horseback had many advantages for traveling through the countryside in those days, especially when it came to negotiating muddy roads or fording rushing streams. But, as he made plans to bring his mother and step-sisters to live with him, he knew that a horse alone would no longer be sufficient. And so he purchased the family buggy—his third mode of transportation—to which he would hitch his faithful old chestnut. This served him well for many years and would always be associated with fond memories of trips into the countryside and moonlit rides with his young wife. Still, it was a new century, and technology was changing the standards of living in many ways, including transportation. Bruce Leslie was not one to be left behind in a changing world and soon transitioned to his fourth mode of transportation.

Throughout most of the nineteenth century, inventors had tinkered with a wide variety of horseless carriages. Toward the end of the century, Karl Benz built a small number of single-cylinder, gasoline-powered automobiles, and the era of "production" vehicles was launched. But the cars that were available around the turn of the century were increasingly elaborate and technically sophisticated and well out of the price range of all but the very wealthy. This changed early in the twentieth century when Henry Ford began experimenting with mass production of automobiles and, in 1908, introduced his Ford Model T, which was affordable for most middle-class Americans, including one Dr. S. B. Leslie.

Blossom was in the kitchen when she heard a peculiar noise in their backyard. At first, she thought it must be a strange bird making a funny honking sound. But then she became concerned when the noise changed to a loud, rumbling racket, and she ran with alarm to the back door to see what could be happening. Out near the barn, the chickens were excitedly scurrying about in their coop, and the old chestnut was nervously stomping his feet and moving from side to side in his stall. And Blossom could only shake her head with an incredulous smile as she watched her husband wrestling a buggy without a horse as it lurched into their backyard.

The two sisters also heard the noise, and before their mother could stop them Elizabeth ran out the back door to discover what it was all about, with Frances doing her best to keep up. When they saw the shiny new automobile with their father sitting proudly behind the wheel, they squealed with delight. Bruce reached down and pulled them up beside him and was about to take them for a ride when Blossom came running out of the house. For a moment, he feared that she might be upset with him, but was then relieved and amused when he saw a smile on her face and the family camera in her hand. And so, with Bruce sitting tall and proud behind the wheel, the two girls on his lap, Blossom took a picture of their family's first car. Also captured in the picture is the old horse, now standing calmly in the barn. One can't help but wonder what he was thinking. That his days of being needed were over? Or that this noisy contraption was just a passing fad and that they would soon be needing him again? Or maybe he was just glad that he would no longer be hauling the family around.

Despite the surprise and excitement of their family's first car that year, Blossom soon had an even more important announcement to make. As the summer of 1913 was coming to an end, she told Bruce and the girls that, come spring of the new year, a new someone special would be joining their family.

The year 1914 would be another time of mixed blessings. For the Leslie family, the blessing came in early April with the arrival of their third daughter (the author's mother), whom they named Ruth Coleman. Like her two older sisters, she too would have her own distinct personality. While Elizabeth was the serious, responsible sister, and Frances the effervescent, irrepressible one, Ruth was more like her mother, with a painful shyness and a delicately tender heart that could break at the least provocation. And, like her namesake of the Old Testament, she would always have a fierce loyalty and devotion to her family. Coincidentally, that same month marked the debut of another Ruth, who pitched his first professional game—Babe Ruth.

With a loving wife, three beautiful, healthy daughters and a busy medical practice, Bruce could only marvel at his blessings, and he never failed to acknowledge his gratitude each day in his prayers. But he was becoming increasingly troubled by world events, especially those taking place in Europe when, in late June, he saw the headlines in the morning paper—*Austrian Archduke Franz Ferdinand Assassinated by Serbian Nationalist.* Bruce knew that this could well be the fuse to ignite a fragile peace in Europe into a major conflagration. And, sadly, his greatest fears would be realized. Within a month, Austria-Hungary declared war on Serbia, launching what would be called the Great War and would one day be known as World War I. One nation after the next took sides in the conflict. German Emperor Wilhelm II declared war on his Russian nephew, Tsar Nicholas II, who reluctantly mobilized his forces. Nicholas was quoted as saying, "Think of the thousands and thousands of men who will be sent to their deaths." Little could he have known then that he and his family would be among the casualties and that events in his country would influence world history for the remainder of the century and beyond.

While Bruce was still no fan of President Wilson, he did appreciate his attempts to keep the United States out of the war. But it was becoming increasingly difficult to maintain a position of neutrality against the German belligerence, especially when, in May of 1915, a U-boat sank the SS *Lusitania* with the loss of 1,198 lives. And yet the United States remained neutral.

Although Bruce worried each day about the war in Europe and the future of his country, he had his own set of problems to deal with on the home front. Blossom had been struggling to care for three young children, when she discovered that their fourth child would be arriving in early winter. Ollie was now married and no longer available to help, and the strain on Blossom was becoming critical. Her parents, who were now living in Colorado Springs, had become increasingly concerned about news they were receiving in letters from their daughter, and they offered a solution. In the spring, when Elizabeth was approaching her sixth birthday, the McKeages came to Okmulgee by train and took their oldest granddaughter to live with them for a while to give Blossom some relief.

Elizabeth's life in Colorado would contain some of her earliest and fondest memories. Every Saturday evening, Grandpa McKeage would walk to the newsstand and buy several papers from major cities and then read the "funnies" to the family. "Tiny Tinies" was her favorite, and she saved copies of those comics to read to her own children many years later. That summer, she celebrated her sixth birthday with her grandparents. And then, in the fall, they received word from Okmulgee that Elizabeth had a little brother, who was christened Samuel Brewster Leslie Jr. and called Sam. While the three girls had their own distinct personalities, they were each unquestionably young ladies, and Sam was all boy. They sent pictures of him and told about all the cute things he did, and Elizabeth desperately wanted to see her little brother. But Blossom, more than ever, needed further time to get her infant son past his first few months. So Elizabeth stayed with her grandparents in Colorado Springs through the Christmas season and into the new year.

She had been gone for nearly a year when her grandparents finally brought her back to Okmulgee. Although Blossom had had little time to think about it with three other children to care for, she had missed Elizabeth terribly and was literally trembling with excitement when the train pulled into the station. But, as Elizabeth stepped down onto the station platform, and Blossom rushed to hug her, she stopped short with an awful realization. Elizabeth had been gone so long that she didn't seem to recognize her mother, and she clung to the skirt of her Grandma McKeage. That was one of the hardest moments she could ever recall. It took some time for mother and daughter to become reattached, and Blossom swore that she would never again let one of her children live away from her.

Elizabeth would always have the most wonderful memories of her time in Colorado, but she had also missed her family terribly. She was amazed to see how much Frances and Ruth had grown during the year she was away, although she was actually the one who had done most of the growing, and all the family marveled at how tall she was. The three young sisters became immediately inseparable and talked incessantly about many things. Most of all they talked about their baby brother, Sam. After three girls in a row, it was something special to now have a little guy in the house with his rough-and-tumble boyish ways that contrasted so strikingly with the dainty manners of his sisters. And what a thrill it was for each of them to be the "big sister" of such a cute little fellow. Most of all, it was just wonderful for the family to be back together again. And yet something seemed to be lacking.

When the time had come for the McKeages to return to Colorado after bringing Elizabeth home, there was considerable sadness. Elizabeth had become closely attached to her grandparents, and they to her, and the thought of their leaving made everyone very sad. And, of course, Blossom had missed her parents greatly during her seven years in Okmulgee and was also dreading the thought of them leaving. All of this did not go unnoticed by Bruce, who began to formulate a plan. Since the loss of Callie, the house next door had sat empty. It was the perfect size for John and Nettie McKeage, and it would be such a joy for everyone to have them all together. And so, the night before they were to return to Colorado, Bruce sat down with his father-in-law for a man-to-man talk.

"Mr. McKeage," he began. (Bruce was always deferential to his elders.) "It looks like you're going to cause a great deal of sadness in my family when you folks leave tomorrow. I've been thinking about that and was wondering if you and Mrs. McKeage might consider moving to Okmulgee. As you know, the house next door is empty, and it would sure be good to have you folks living beside us. I know it would make all my family awfully happy."

Bruce was not given to excessive chatter, and he stopped at that point to give his father-in-law time to consider his proposal (which, in truth, he had also been ruminating about). John McKeage was also a man of few words, and the two men sat quietly for several minutes in their own thoughts. Then John nodded his head and said, "I'll discuss it with Nettie."

They all went to the train station the following morning to say goodbye, and there were hugs and tears all around. No one knew for sure what the future might hold for their families. But the McKeages had not been back in Colorado Springs long before Bruce received a letter from John stating that he and Nettie had decided to accept his kind offer and that they planned to move to Okmulgee early in the new year. Needless to say, Elizabeth and her mother were overjoyed to receive such wonderful news, as were the other children, who had also quickly grown to love their grandparents.

And so 1916 ended with much joy and thanksgiving in the Leslie family. Bruce and Blossom now had four beautiful and healthy children, and they were all together in their warm, comfortable home. And, like icing on the cake, Blossom's parents would be coming to live with them in a matter of months. The only thing that cast a shadow over the year was the bloody conflict that continued to rage in Europe and the fear that the United States might soon be drawn into it. Three weeks after his re-election, President Wilson had declared an end to his neutrality policy, and the nation held its collective breath to see what the new year would hold.

And, indeed, 1917 had an ominous beginning. Germany notified America that their submarines would be attacking neutral merchant ships, and in February the S.S. *Housatonic* was sunk by a U-boat. Wilson broke diplomatic relations with Germany, and the country finally began to prepare for war. But John and Nettie McKeage kept to their plans and moved to Okmulgee in the spring. Blossom's brother Charlie came with them, although he soon left to join the Army as a sharpshooter. He had always been an excellent marksman and hoped to join General Pershing's American Expeditionary Force, which was planning to sail for France that spring. All his family, of course, prayed that he would not be put in harm's way, and it turned out that their prayers were answered. To Charlie's disappointment and embarrassment, he remained stationed in the United States for the remainder of the war, and many prayers of thanks went up for that blessing.

The year ended with the United States declaring war on Austria and becoming a full-fledged participant in the Great War. Of lesser note, to many people at least, Congress approved the Eighteenth Amendment, which led to the prohibition of alcohol and would have major consequences on the country in the years that lay ahead. At forty-four years of age, Bruce Leslie did not join the military, but he proved to be an important "soldier" at home, facing a worldwide killer that was even more deadly than the war.

In the summer of 1918, Bruce was just finishing a long day of clinic visits and house calls when a young boy came into his office. He wore ragged, dirty clothes and was obviously exhausted and in a state of near panic. He reported to the doctor that his father was "real sick" and that his mother had finally told him to go for help. They were sharecroppers who lived on a small plot of land in the county. The boy had apparently run all the way to get help for his father. Dr. Leslie listened to his story and realized that he needed to get out there quickly. He and the boy walked briskly to the Leslie homestead, where they got into the Model T and headed out into the country.

The house they pulled up to was small and rundown, and it was apparent that hygiene was not a high priority for the family. As he stepped inside, Bruce was accosted by a variety of unpleasant odors, but one was of particular concern to him. He had learned to recognize the smells of different diseases and, even before examining his patient, he knew what he was dealing with. Sure enough, the young man was lying on a dirty bed struggling to breathe. Although it was the first case of this viral strain that he had seen, Bruce knew immediately that his patient had influenza. The first cases had been reported in the spring and had now spread around the world. By that fall, the flu would reportedly take 21,000 lives in the United States in a single week, with a final estimate of 700,000 at home and millions worldwide. Even these numbers were probably underestimates. All the countries engaged in the Great War, including the United States, were underreporting their cases in order to maintain morale at home for the war effort. But Spain remained neutral and had no reason not to report accurate numbers, making it appear that the prevalence in that country was higher and giving rise to the pandemic's nickname— Spanish flu.

Bruce knew that the flu primarily afflicted young adults and that malnutrition and poor hygiene were associated with the higher rate of mortality from the illness. He did all he could to make his patient comfortable, but it was too late. The young man had been sick in bed for several days before the family sought medical care, and he died the following evening. But Bruce knew that the number of deaths in his community could be minimized by isolating all future cases and by encouraging good hygiene and nutrition, as well as wearing masks and maintaining social distances. And it was largely thanks to the tireless efforts of Dr. Leslie and the medical community that Okmulgee was spared the major devastation of the Influenza of 1918.

One morning that summer, Bruce picked up the newspaper and shook his head in despair to read that the new Bolshevik government in Russia had executed Tsar Nicholas and his entire family. He could not help but wonder what effect this would have on world affairs as the century continued to unfold. The news, however, was not all bad that year. Blossom was pleased to read that the House of Representatives had passed an amendment for women's suffrage, and Bruce shared her pleasure. But the most encouraging news of all came that fall, with the dissolution of the Austro-Hungarian Empire and the abdication of Emperor Wilhelm, who fled to the Netherlands. And then, on November eleventh, an armistice was signed between the Allies and Germany, effectively ending the Great War.

Christmas 1918 was an especially joyful time for the Leslie family. The war was over. Their four children were healthy and happy. Blossom's parents were now living next door, and Charlie had returned home safely and was also living with them. The adults all sat back comfortably in the warmth of the family room with a contented smile on each face. As the lights twinkled on the fragrant tree, Bruce looked around at all his blessings. Baby Sam was in his mother's arms, and the three girls were playing on the floor with their newly acquired treasures. He took it all in and had no doubt that the room was filled with God's grace. He closed his eyes for a brief moment and said a prayer of profound thanks.

CHAPTER 10

Faith and Justice

"MAMA, FRANCIE HAS BEEN IN THE BATHROOM all morning!"

"Frances, let Elizabeth in. We've got to share, and it's getting late."

"Mama, what shall I wear?"

"I ironed your yellow dress this morning, Ruth. It's hanging in your closet."

"Mama, I'm too tired to get up!"

"You've had plenty of sleep, Samuel. Now hop up and let's get you dressed."

Such was the banter on a typical Sunday morning, as Blossom struggled to get her four children ready for church. She had risen before dawn on this spring day, cooking, ironing, laying out clothes and then getting them all up. The girls were now old enough to dress themselves, but little Sam still required close attention. When they had all been younger, she was often so exhausted after getting everyone else ready that she didn't have enough energy left to dress herself and go to church. But, on this Sunday, she looked forward to joining the family because a guest pastor of some note was scheduled to preach and, more importantly, her husband would be giving his last Sunday School lesson for awhile.

Bruce Leslie had also risen before dawn and walked downtown to his office to put the final touches on the lesson he would be giving later that morning. From the day he joined the Methodist Church of Okmulgee, just after moving there in 1902, he had been one of its most active members. Back when he first joined, it was called the Methodist Episcopal Church South, and the congregation was a congenial blend of Creek Indians, whites, and a few Black members. But circumstances in Okmulgee had changed over the years, and the composition of the church, which was now simply called the Methodist Church, had gradually become increasingly white. Bruce regretted this change, but remained loyal to his church throughout his life, doing whatever he could to nurture it both physically and spiritually.

He had begun teaching an adult Sunday School class shortly after joining the church and before long was serving on their planning board. In 1910, he helped oversee the construction of a new church building to which he contributed substantially from his personal resources. In all, he helped finance three new buildings for his church and donated two five-room bungalows for retired ministers. He also contributed to the growth of other churches in town and would eventually devote much of his attention to a small country church just outside of Okmulgee. But on this early Sunday morning he was preparing the Sunday School lesson that would be his last for awhile. He was temporarily stepping down from his teaching role because he was about to take over as superintendent of all the Sunday School classes in his Methodist Church, a position he would hold for many years.

Blossom and the children were dressed and waiting when their father returned home. He stood and looked at them for a moment, as if inspecting the troops, and then announced with a smile that it was the handsomest family he had ever seen. He was never given to excessive displays of affection, but no one in the family ever doubted that he loved them more than anything in the world. After giving each child a little pat, he went out to warm up their new car.

His first Model T Ford hadn't lasted long. For one thing, it required a crank to manually start the engine, which was not always cooperative. Especially on cold nights, when he had to get up to make a house call, it could be frustratingly contrary. He frequently had to boil water to pour over the engine to warm it up before it would start. Another disadvantage was that it only had a front seat, which was not nearly enough room for his now large family of six. So he traded in the "tin Lizzie," as they were colloquially known, for a newer and larger Ford, which was soon purring nicely on that Sunday morning as his family piled in and headed off to church.

A large group had already gathered in his Sunday School classroom when the family arrived. The children went to their respective classes, and Blossom joined her husband in his class. As had been the case when he lived in Denver, Bruce was a very popular teacher. In fact, it happened to be Pentecostal Sunday, and the lesson he had prepared was a revision of a lesson that he had once given on that subject when he taught the young ladies' class in Denver.

"We can now look at Pentecost as one of the most important days of the world," he began after an opening prayer. "The coming of the Holy Ghost was accompanied by three signs: wind, fire, and tongues." As he spoke of the metaphorical meaning of wind, his mind may have drifted back to a time, just after the loss of his father, when he had first sensed the powerful presence of God in a breeze whirling about his head. It was a feeling that he would experience many times in his life. He likened it to the power of wind over the ocean that drives a sailing ship—a power that cannot be seen, but the effect of which is clearly visible. He spoke of the fire as "a warm spirit in all our work," by which he meant the energy that drives us to make the most of the talents with which we are blessed. "We badly need this fire in our church and school," he said with a clear sense of urgency. And he spoke of the symbol of tongues as an admonition to spread God's message of love in word and deed: "We have more to do than to be worshippers and believers." And with those final words, he was likely thinking of one of his favorite Bible verses from the book of James, "Be ye doers of the word and not hearers only."

After the closing prayer, everyone got up and enjoyed a brief time of fellowship—an opportunity to chat with their teacher and catch up with friends on what was happening in the community— before moving into the sanctuary for the morning worship service. The guest speaker lived up to his billing, although Blossom felt she got more out of her husband's lesson. In any case, she and Bruce joined the other parishioners at the end of the service as they filed out through the front door to greet and shake hands with the guest preacher. When it came Blossom's turn, she complimented him on his sermon and said she hoped to meet him again one day. Little did she know how soon that day would be.

When they got home, Blossom went upstairs and changed into her working clothes before starting their Sunday dinner. She had just come back down and entered the kitchen when she heard a knock at the front door. It was then that Bruce remembered something he had forgotten to tell her (one of Blossom's pet peeves about her husband). He had invited the guest preacher to have dinner with them. She was not about to let their guest see her in her work clothes, but in order to get upstairs to change, she would have to go through the living room, where the two men were chatting. So she quickly devised a plan. Elizabeth was helping her in the kitchen, and Blossom gave her daughter some paper and string and told her to wrap her Sunday clothes in the paper and lower it down from an upstairs window to the kitchen window below. Elizabeth did as she was instructed, and her mother retrieved the package, changed back into her Sunday clothes in the kitchen and came out to graciously welcome their guest.

During their dinner, the preacher complimented Blossom on a delicious meal and then mercifully departed shortly after dessert and coffee. She went back upstairs and again changed into her work clothes, came down and washed the dishes, and finally went to the living room to collapse. Bruce was resting there in his easy chair, reading the Sunday paper. Blossom was exhausted and thankful to have a moment of peace. And a moment is about what it was. She had no sooner sat down than all four children came to her. Elizabeth and Frances needed help with their homework, Ruth was having a problem with a doll dress she was working on, and little Sam just wanted someone to play with him. Blossom looked over hopefully at Bruce, but saw that he was fast asleep with the paper in his lap. She knew better than to wake him, because his demanding medical practice required that he get all the sleep he could whenever he could. And so, with a sigh and a weary smile, Blossom was reminded once again of the old adage: "A man can work from sun to sun, but a woman's work is never done."

If Blossom ever felt put upon by the role she played in her family, she never spoke of it. But there were many women around the world who had been vocal for over a century about gender inequity in politics, business, and society in general. It was not until the mid-nineteenth century that some countries began to grant women's suffrage (often to rescind it later). The Great War may have contributed to their cause by showing, during the war effort, that women were quite capable of making major contributions to their communities. In any case, Canada granted women the right to vote in 1917, and England and Germany did the same the following year. Then, in June of 1919, the U.S. Congress passed the Woman's Suffrage Bill as the Nineteenth Amendment, although it still required ratification.

Blossom was a charter member of the TNT club, which stood for "Thimble, Needle, and Thread." That name would later be a source of embarrassment for the ladies of the club when the initials became commonly associated with the explosive. But in 1920 it was a peaceful gathering of women who enjoyed stitching, chatting, and each other's company. The two main topics of conversation in those days were prohibition and ratification of the Nineteenth Amendment. The former had gone into effect in January, much to the approval of the women, and they now focused most of their conversations on the suffrage issue. Blossom rarely entered into those discussions. She obviously wanted what was best for women, but she had grown up in a family where a woman's place was felt to be in the home, and she was content to leave certain responsibilities to the men. Nevertheless, in August of that year, when one of the women came bursting into the house where the TNT ladies were gathered, and waved the morning paper with the headline *U.S. Ratifies 19th Amendment*, Blossom celebrated cheerfully with the rest of them.

The news of the day was also a major topic of conversation for the Leslie family as they sat around the dinner table each evening. Their father had told his family, earlier in the year, that he favored the concept of prohibition but feared the consequences it would likely have for the country. And already an increase in crime was being reported. That summer, he also expressed his pleasure that women would now have the right to vote, which he agreed was long overdue. But the one event that won his unequivocal approval in the fall of that year was the election of Warren G. Harding as the 29th president. Frankly, Bruce didn't think too much of Harding as an individual but was just relieved to have the administration back in the hands of the Republicans. And so 1920 came to an end with the country divided over the major events of the year, leaving many people happy and others disgruntled.

Ruth had never before seen her father cry. She had just walked into the living room and found him sitting alone with a newspaper in his lap and tears in his eyes. It was unsettling to her sensitive temperament, and she didn't quite know what to do. Her father had always been the strength in her life—the one who gave her comfort when she felt like crying—the one who taught her not to cry but to look for solutions to her problems. But, despite such teachings, she had a very tender heart and now, finding herself alone with her distraught father, the tears began to flow down her own cheeks, although she had no idea why. She walked quietly to his side and put her hand on his arm. This startled him and caused the newspaper to fall from his lap. And then she saw the headline: *Hundreds killed in Tulsa Massacre.*

When the Creek Indians, especially those of mixed-race, had been forced to leave their ancestral homes along the East Coast and move to Indian Territory in the 1830s, some brought their Black slaves with them. After the Civil War, many of the freed Blacks joined the Creek Nation and became known as Freedmen. Toward the end of the nineteenth century, when Bruce Leslie had come there as a traveling salesman, an increasing number of white settlers were being allowed to purchase land in the area. He found that everyone seemed to coexist reasonably well in those days and that this was still pretty much the case when he returned in 1902—Indians, Blacks, and whites did business together, went to the same schools, worshipped together, and often intermarried.

But all this began to change as more whites, especially from the Deep South, moved into the area with their Jim Crow laws. And then in 1907, with Oklahoma statehood and loss of tribal autonomy, the federal government required that schools be segregated. Many Indians sold their land and moved west. The growing number of whites took over the businesses in the center of Okmulgee, and the Blacks were pushed to the north and east sides of town. They now had their own churches, and the Methodist Church and other mainstream churches in Okmulgee became increasingly white.

These changes were of great concern to Dr. Leslie. His interpretation of the Bible was that we are all equal in God's eyes and that we should love each other and try to live in harmony. But others in Okmulgee, including some church leaders, interpreted the Bible differently. They somehow felt that separation of Blacks and whites was part of the natural order and that, even though they might not admit it, white privilege was a part of that order. Bruce soon realized that this was the majority (if unspoken) view among the white citizens of Okmulgee and that he was in an ever-shrinking minority. And this created a practical problem for him during the early days, as he was getting his practice started, because he felt an obligation to provide equal medical care for all the citizens of his community.

It had never occurred to Bruce that all his patients shouldn't sit together in the same waiting room. During his first six months in Arlington House, it hadn't been much of a problem, since the waiting room was just the foyer, and patients could also wait outside on the porch if they chose. But when he moved his office to the Bank of Commerce building, where he had a proper waiting room and a much larger practice, some of his more vocal white patients began to complain that they were not comfortable sitting in the same room with a Black person. This had created a serious conundrum for the young doctor, who only wanted to be fair to everyone. Then one day a solution to the problem seemed to come in a most unexpected way.

It was a Saturday morning, shortly after Bruce had moved to his new office. He had gone there to catch up on some paperwork and was surprised to find a young Black man waiting for him on the upstairs landing just outside his office. He was in obvious pain and leaning on a homemade crutch. Bruce did not hold regular clinics on Saturdays in those early days, but he could see that the young man needed his immediate attention, so he asked him to come into his office. The man introduced himself as Jeremiah and said that he had a small farm just outside of town. He had been plowing behind a mule when he turned his leg in one of the furrows. At first, he thought it was just a bad sprain, but it hadn't gotten any better after a week, and he couldn't put any weight on the leg. A quick examination revealed an obvious fracture, and the doctor marveled that his patient had made it to his office, especially when he learned that he had walked all the way, with the help of his makeshift crutch. He was able to reduce the fracture and then put a splint on the leg. But he couldn't imagine how Jeremiah could get back home on his own, so he told him to wait while he went to his house and got his horse and buggy.

When they got to Jeremiah's home, Bruce's heart ached to see what a pitiful shack it was. But Jeremiah seemed proud of it and invited the doctor to come up on the porch for something to drink. The two men were about the same age, but Jeremiah was already married with three children, and he was proud to introduce his family to the doctor. As the two men sat on the porch, Jeremiah's wife brought them both a glass of sweet tea, and Bruce enjoyed his chat with Jeremiah. He was especially pleased to learn more about the farmland around Okmulgee, a subject that was becoming of increased interest to him.

Dr. Leslie saw Jeremiah several times for follow-up visits, but always on Saturday mornings at his patient's request. One day, when Bruce suggested another day of the week for his next visit, Jeremiah was silent for a moment and seemed embarrassed by what he was about to say.

"Doctuh Leslie, suh, if'n you don't mind, I rathuh not come when the white folks is there."

This surprised Bruce. It had never occurred to him that his Black patients might feel just as uncomfortable as the whites sitting together. Jeremiah said he was pretty sure that this was how most of the Black folks felt. And that's when a solution to the doctor's problem seemed to present itself. Saturday mornings were a good time for his Black patients to be seen, because that is when they could most easily get off work and when they came into town. And so Bruce started a regular Saturday morning clinic for them, and it worked well for many years.

But there was another matter that was also bothering Jeremiah. Dr. Leslie had not said anything to him about payment for all the time and care he had given him. One Saturday morning, he brought a one-dollar bill with him in the hope of beginning to cover his medical expenses. Bruce had a pretty good idea what this money meant to his family. It probably meant less food on the table. He had been thinking about this for awhile and felt that now was a good time to discuss it.

"Jeremiah, I understand you have a barbershop over on the east side," he began.

"Yes suh, I do cuts some folks' hair a few days a week," Jeremiah responded.

"Would you be willing to take me as a customer?"

This took his patient totally by surprise. "You would come to my shop, suh?"

"Well, I have to get my hair cut somewhere, and I think that should make us even on your medical expenses and for whatever care you and your family might need in the future."

Bruce saw tears beginning to well up in Jeremiah's eyes and hoped he had done the right thing. But the two men agreed to the arrangement and, for years to come, that would be how Dr. Leslie got his haircuts.

Over the years that followed, Bruce enjoyed a congenial relationship with his Black patients, seeing them in his Saturday morning clinics, visiting them on their farms, and walking over to the east side for his haircuts. But he did this at a price. The majority of white people in Okmulgee observed strict segregation, and Bruce knew that some people talked about him behind his back. He wasn't bothered by that. What did bother him deeply, however, was news of race riots, in which Blacks were being killed and their property destroyed by groups of white people. In the "Red Summer" of 1919, this happened in several dozen cities around the country.

Bruce could not understand why some white people seemed to hate their black neighbors so intensely. What had they ever done to them? But these events had occurred in other states, and he found some consolation in the belief (or hope) that Oklahomans were above such treachery—that is, until he opened his newspaper in early June of 1921.

Because the territory had enjoyed reasonable racial harmony, especially before statehood, Oklahoma became known as a place where persons of all heritages could come for a chance to realize the American dream. As a result, many prominent Black families moved to Tulsa, which is about thirty miles from Okmulgee. They developed a neighborhood called the Greenwood district. Its doctors and lawyers and entrepreneurs created such a prosperous community that it was often referred to as "Black Wall Street." But on May 31, 1921 a large group of angry whites, enraged by a minor misunderstanding, stormed the district, killing the citizens and burning down their homes, buildings, and churches. When it was all over, approximately 300 Black citizens were dead, and their community was destroyed.

That was the news that had brought her father to tears when Ruth found him alone that day in the living room. She continued to cry with him, as she stood by his side, although she still had no idea why they were crying. He smiled and quietly tried to comfort her, but it was too much to grasp for a tender child of seven years. It would be many years later before she would fully understand what had happened that day or appreciate the depth of her father's character.

$\gamma\cdot\lambda$

The 1920s were a time of prosperity for the country, and Okmulgee was no exception. Oil, coal, and cotton were bringing high prices, and railroads were exporting the local products as the economy boomed. Okmulgee was said to have more millionaires during those years than any town of comparable size. It was the golden age of vaudeville, and several theaters in town, such as the Hippodrome, boasted traveling shows and competed with each other. And there were amusement parks, such as Douglas Park and Lambert's Amusement Park, with rides and games and pleasure boats that glided along small lagoons.

For the Leslie children, it was a great time and place to grow up. They enjoyed the shows and the parks as well as the many natural amenities that the area had to offer. Okmulgee Creek flowed by just across the street from their home and provided a pleasant spot to sit on the bank and fish on warm summer days. (Unfortunately, in years to come, pollution would render the creek less attractive and off limits to the grandchildren, when it was commonly known as Greasy Creek.)

Their father liked to have the children go with him when he drove out into the country to make house calls or visit farms. And, for the most part, they enjoyed it also, especially when they got to make special stops along the way. For example, in early summer, when wild blackberries were ripe, they would stop and pick them, knowing what delicious cobblers their mother would make. These times occasionally also had their humorous, if not frightening, moments. On one occasion, the vines had grown up into the trees and, as Frances reached up for some berries, she found herself eye to eye with a snake. She screamed and ran, which her Daddy thought was quite amusing. He grabbed the snake by the tail and swung it around to break its "neck." But it slipped out of his hand and wound around Frances's neck. It was already dead by this time and immediately slipped off the terrified child, but it was some time before she and her three siblings could stop screaming and jumping up and down.

In those days, no houses had central heating, which posed a problem in the Leslie household during the cold days of winter. Their single bathroom upstairs had a small heater that didn't keep it very warm. The kitchen was the warmest room in the house, and on Saturday nights during the winter, Blossom would set up a large metal tub in the kitchen and fill it with hot water so that each child could take a turn bathing. It may have been a bit like a party for the three sisters, but poor little Sam, being the youngest and the only boy, saw it quite differently. Even at his young age, he was modest enough to insist, "Make those girls get out of here!" when it was his turn to bathe.

Another measure for conserving heat in the house during the winter was the heavy velvet curtains that separated the living room from the dining room. This kept the living room a bit warmer so that the family could sit together on cold nights to read or play games, such as Whist, which was one of their favorites. When it was time for bed, the children would all gather in the larger bedroom that Frances and Ruth shared, and their parents would take turns reading to them. Among their favorite books were *Trail of the Lonesome Pine* and *Who's Your School Master*. Then they would say their prayers together, and their parents would tuck each child in bed under a mound of blankets and sit on the edge of the bed for a moment as cobwebs began to fill the children's heads.

On some nights, it was more difficult for the children to drift off to sleep, especially when something was troubling them and they needed to talk. One night, when Ruth was eight years old, she told her Daddy that she had been thinking about the stories he told them of his time in Denver and that it was making her sad.

"Weren't you afraid and lonely to be in such a big town?" she asked.

"Well, I did have a friend with me," he replied with a smile. "I had Jesus."

And that seemed to satisfy Ruth, who said "good night" and turned over into her pillow.

On another night, it was Frances who seemed upset about something. It was a Sunday, and her father noticed that she had appeared a bit pensive ever since returning home from church.

"Daddy, am I saved?" she asked.

Her father smiled and assured her that she was, although he suspected that something deeper was bothering her.

"But I don't think I want to be saved," she almost whispered with a growing frown.

Bruce knew Frances's Sunday School teacher. She was a good teacher, but tended to adhere to rather fundamental interpretations of the Bible, which he feared was the source of his daughter's disquietude. And yet he felt that he should let her explain, so he simply responded with a quizzical look.

"Our Sunday School teacher told us that Jesus had to die so God would forgive us for being bad, and so we would be saved and get to go to heaven."

She had been thinking about that all day, and it upset her, because she couldn't understand why it had to be that way. Her father nodded sympathetically, as though to say "Please tell me more."

"Can't God do whatever he wants?" she wondered. "And couldn't he forgive me and let me go to heaven without having to make poor Jesus get killed?"

Her father took a deep breath and gave his daughter another quiet smile. It was a mystery that he had pondered over the years, and he was amazed that such a young child could also wonder about it and articulate it so clearly. The question, to his mind, was whether Jesus died to change God's mind about us or to change our minds about God. He had come to believe that it was the latter and thought for a moment about how to phrase it in appropriate words for a child.

"Frances," he began softly. "I think Jesus died to teach us all something very important. I believe that God loves you so very much and that he let Jesus die to show you just how much you are loved. What greater love could there be than that? And when someone loves you that much, you want to love them back. I know you love Jesus. And because you love him, maybe that's what it means to be saved, because you live in God's love now and you will forever."

Frances looked up into her father's gentle hazel eyes and did her best to comprehend what he had just told her. Then, with a serious look on her face, she nodded her understanding, closed her eyes and, as her lips relaxed into a serene smile, she drifted off into peaceful slumber.

On a hot summer day in early August of 1923, Bruce Leslie opened up his morning newspaper to find startling headlines. President Harding had died of a heart attack while on a tour of the Western States. The news caused a wave of sorrow to suddenly wash over the doctor. It was not so much for the president or his family as it was for the country, which was now in mourning. Harding had been enjoying a high level of national popularity at the time, although Bruce had reservations about his character. And his concerns would be justified, when corruption and scandal in Harding's administration, as well as the president's personal improprieties, would eventually come to light.

Calvin Coolidge had been quickly sworn in as the thirtieth president and, even though he vowed to continue Harding's policies and retain his cabinet, Bruce had a feeling that the country was now in better hands. And time would also support that opinion. One of the achievements that especially pleased Dr. Leslie was the Indian Citizenship Act, which Coolidge signed into law in June of the following year. Bruce felt passionately about equal rights for all people, not only for women and persons of African heritage, but also for the indigenous Americans, who had been so badly treated by his government. He hoped that this latest act of Congress, which gave U.S. citizenship to all American Indians, would be a meaningful step toward beginning to right those wrongs. In any case, he looked forward to discussing it with his old friend Amos McIntosh.

Amos still ran the general store downtown, but he now had a teenage son, Amos Jr., who worked part-time to help his father. It was approaching closing time when Bruce walked into the store and was warmly greeted by the senior McIntosh. This was not an uncommon meeting for the two friends, who had now known each other for a couple of decades. Over those years, Bruce had learned a great deal about the McIntosh clan and the Creek Nation and how both had become an integral part of Okmulgee history.

In 1735, John McIntosh and his wife, Margaret, sailed from Scotland with their two sons and a group of Scottish Highlanders, setting ashore on the banks of Savannah, Georgia. There were already a few fellow Scottish families living in the area. Some had come over directly from Scotland, while others had moved to Ireland for a generation or more before migrating to the New World. The Scots lived among the indigenous people of the Creek Nation, and it was not uncommon for them to marry into Creek families, especially those of the Lower Creek division, which was friendlier with the white settlers. One of the McIntosh boys, William, married a comely young Creek tribal maiden by the name of Senoya, who was of the privileged, aristocratic Wind Clan. They prospered, building a plantation and owning many African slaves. In 1778, William and Senoya were blessed with a son, William Jr. The young man grew in stature, bridging the two cultures into which he was born and eventually becoming Chief William McIntosh Jr., Chief of the Lower Creeks.

Chief William married a woman named Eliza, who was also of mixed Scottish and Creek heritage, and she gave birth to their first child at the turn of the century. They named him Chilly. When he grew older, the boy often traveled with his father and learned leadership traits from him. One day, they rode beside the bank of a river that bordered on land which the Creeks were negotiating with the new white government. His father explained that the name of the river in Creek meant "bubbling water" and was pronounced Okmulgee.

The story at this point goes from one tragedy to another. The U.S. government continued to usurp land from the Creeks, until the Treaty of 1825 in which Chief William signed off on all their remaining land in Georgia in return for land to the west of the Mississippi River. The Upper Creeks, also known as "Red Sticks," were furious with William, and a band of them came to his plantation home, dragged him out on the front lawn, murdered him, and burned down the house. Chilly saw it all from a distance and barely escaped with his own life.

By now, Chilly was married with a young family and had become Chief Chilly McIntosh, leader of one of the Lower Creek tribes. He recognized that there was no longer any future for his people in their ancient land and began to organize voluntary migrations west to land that the government had designated as "Indian Territory." Over the years that followed, Chief Chilly led many groups into the land that would eventually become known as Arkansas and Oklahoma. In 1842, he and fellow Creek leaders hosted a Grand Council beside a winding river, called the Deep Fork, in which water bubbled over the rock-strewn bed. It may have reminded Chilly of the river that he and his father once rode beside in Georgia. In any case, they gave the river the Creek name for "bubbling water," and eventually gave the same name to the location where they had sat in council and which would one day become the capital of the Creek Nation—Okmulgee.

Bruce had heard the story many times and knew most of it by heart. He also knew that the misfortunes of the Native Americans had not stopped with their arrival in Indian Territory. The federal government had promised autonomy for Creeks and other tribal nations in their new land, but even that was taken from them when Oklahoma became a state in 1907. In addition to Amos, Bruce had many friends among the Creeks, most of whom were his patients, and it embarrassed and saddened him that his people were treating the Indians this way. It was for this reason that he had been heartened to read the news that morning of U.S. citizenship for all American Indians. He hoped that this might be the beginning of a better relationship between the two cultures. In any case, as the two old friends sat down in the back of the store for a chat, Bruce was interested in Amos's take on it.

"Yes," Amos began, "it is an encouraging step. But I'm not sure what it really means for my people. You may have noticed, Bruce, that the act does not include voting rights for Indians. That will be left up to each state, and it remains to be seen what Oklahoma will do."

Bruce remained silent, listening intently to his friend's thoughts.

Amos went on, "My distant relatives in Georgia felt that our best hope was to cooperate with the whites and try to assimilate among them. But you see where that got us. We are trying to do that again here in Oklahoma. Some of us have succeeded reasonably well, but many of my people continue to struggle. I'm not sure that the white people trust us. It's hard for Indians to get decent jobs or to have the whites trade with us. So many become depressed and turn to drinking."

This was obviously not the upbeat conversation that Bruce was hoping to have with Amos, but he appreciated his friend's frankness. And Amos could see the worry in Bruce's eyes and knew what he was thinking, without him saying a word: *What can I do to help?*

"Bruce, you are doing so much in our community to help my people," Amos resumed talking, after a long pause. "The medical care you give so many of us would be more than enough. And you treat us all as equals and never worry about how we pay you."

Bruce did not do well with compliments. He was beginning to blush and wish they could change the subject, but Amos continued.

"One of the most important ways to help my people is through education, and who is doing more for that in Okmulgee than you.

Your role as chairman of the school board and all you have done to create new schools in our town is one of the best hopes we have for our children to succeed in the next generation."

Now Bruce was really becoming uncomfortable with the praise. That wasn't what he had come to talk about. But Amos was right. Although Dr. Leslie may not have fully recognized it, or just chose not to talk about it, his contributions to their community were increasing every year and were clearly making life better for all segments of the society. But, of all his contributions, the one for which Bruce was most passionate was his work in the church. Amos knew that and couldn't drop the line of conversation without including it.

"Your Sunday School lessons have meant so much to many of us, and now with your role as superintendent of the Sunday School department, you are touching an even larger number of people at the Methodist Church. And the work you have done to provide new buildings, not only for the Methodists, but other denominations in town, continues to expand your reach."

Bruce had now had enough. He appreciated his friend's kind words and told him so, but he desperately wanted to change the topic of conversation away from himself. So, before Amos could get started again, Bruce quickly asked him how the family was doing.

"Everyone is doing well, thanks. Amos Jr. has been a big help in the store. Which reminds me; we had a farmer come in the other day who told us about a church they are trying to start, or keep going, somewhere out north of town. I think he called it something like Grovania."

The doctor had never heard the name, but was intrigued by it, wondering what it meant. He would have been even more intrigued if he could have known then what the name and the church would one day mean to him.

As was their custom, the two friends said a prayer together before parting. On that day, Amos offered to recite the first lines of an ancient Indian Prayer:

"O Great Spirit, whose voice I hear in the winds, and whose breath gives life to all the world, hear me! I am small and weak, I need your strength and wisdom."

And the two old friends said in unison, "Amen."

1924 came to a pleasant conclusion for the Leslie family, with Calvin Coolidge defeating John Davis for his full term as U.S. president. But 1925 offered omens of things to come, with the death of Lenin in Russia and the ensuing battle for power between Stalin and Trotsky. And in Munich, Germany, a man by the name of Hitler, who had recently been released from prison after a conviction of treason, had resurrected the Nazi Party.

But the news that interested Bruce Leslie the most that year was the conviction in July of John Scopes, who was convicted for teaching evolution in the Tennessee public school system, a practice that had been outlawed by the governor earlier that year. The heated debate over evolution and the question of religion versus science puzzled Bruce. He could never understand why some people felt that the two were incompatible, and yet he always tried to respect the opinions and beliefs of all individuals.

A footnote to 1925 was the opening of the Okmulgee Country Club and Golf Course. It was for whites only. Needless to say, Bruce Leslie did not care to join.

CHAPTER 11

Education, Land, and the Depression

I

T WAS EARLY SEPTEMBER 1926 and the Leslie children's first day back at school. The family were all gathered around the dining room table for their evening repast, and their father opened the mealtime conversation, as was their custom, with a question.

"What did your teacher talk about in school today?" he directed at no child in particular.

The question was one that their father often asked them, and it led to a frequent topic of dinnertime conversation: the children's education. It was a subject of keen interest to Bruce Leslie for at least two reasons. First, having been limited to rudimentary formal training as a youth himself, he wanted to ensure that his children received the best education possible. And second, as president of the Okmulgee Board of Education, he wanted to know how the school policies that he had helped put in place were working.

The four children looked at each other, wondering who should be the first to address their father's question. Finally, Ruth spoke up.

"My teacher asked where we went on vacation," she offered.

There followed a moment of silence, as all eyes turned toward Ruth to learn how she had responded to her teacher's query.

"I told them we didn't go anywhere."

At that, the children all diverted their gazes down at their plates, and Blossom cast an accusatory glance toward her husband, who immediately felt the heat. The truth was that, aside from their honeymoon, Bruce had never taken a real vacation. He had always been so busy with his host of responsibilities that a family vacation had yet to make the cut. For more than a decade, Blossom had repeatedly pointed out to him that they were missing golden opportunities for the family to enjoy traveling together, with all the interactions, experiences, and memories that come with it. And now that the children were entering their teens, the window for that opportunity was starting to close. Bruce always agreed with Blossom and promised her that they would do it "next summer," although it had yet to happen. But Ruth's comment that evening caused her father to feel the full weight of his shortcoming, and he vowed to himself at that moment to make amends. Come next summer, he would take his family on a real vacation.

As fall faded into winter, Bruce continued his hectic schedule, which included his responsibilities on the school board. He had first been elected to the board back in 1910, the year that Blossom gave birth to their first child. At that time, there were only 800 pupils and three buildings in the Okmulgee city school system. He had worked hard to improve the standards of education for the city, first by serving on committees for finance, auditing, and teachers. Then, in his fifth year, he was elected president of the board, an office he would hold for the next sixteen years. By 1922, Okmulgee boasted two high school buildings and six modern grade schools that accommodated over 5,000 students. The board met twice each month, and during his first 12 years, as an example of his dedication, he missed only two meetings, despite his medical practice and all his other obligations.

One of his duties as president of the board was to recruit well-qualified individuals to serve as teachers and administrators in the city's school system. On several occasions, Bruce traveled to other states to interview and secure the very best he could find for these positions. As a testament to his judgement and recruiting skills, two of the people he hired later moved on to become nationally prominent educators. Dr. H. B. Bruner served as superintendent of the Okmulgee school system and then was associated with Columbia University in New York City before taking the role of superintendent of schools for the city of Minneapolis. Dr. Eugene Briggs also served as a top official in Okmulgee's school administration and later moved to Enid, Oklahoma, as president of Phillips University, where two of the Leslies' grandsons would later matriculate.

Christmas came, and Bruce had not forgotten his personal vow to take the family on a vacation in the coming summer. During the holiday break, he announced that, when school let out for the summer, they would be going on a special trip—their first family vacation. Of course, the children were ecstatic, and Blossom was pleased. But their enthusiasm was tempered somewhat when Bruce shared the details with them. The children, of course, had dreamed of exotic resorts with lakes, mountains, and adventures. Their father, however, being both frugal and a family man, informed them that they would be visiting relatives. It was the beginning of a family tradition of summer vacations, most of which would be to Leslie, Arkansas, where Uncle Andrew and Uncle John still lived with their families. But their first family trip would be a bit more exciting. They would be driving to visit Bruce's sister, Floy, and her family in the Black Hills of South Dakota.

The time between Christmas and summer seemed like an eternity for the Leslie children but flew by for their parents. Bruce continued to be occupied with his many responsibilities, including his role on the school board. In the spring, the Oklahoma State Boards of Education held their first conference in conjunction with the sixteenth annual convention of the Oklahoma Education Association. The joint meeting took place in Oklahoma City, and the delegate from Okmulgee, Dr. S. B. Leslie, had the distinction of being elected to serve as vice-president of the Oklahoma State Boards of Education.

Later that spring, Bruce attended the commencement exercises of Okmulgee High School, as was his custom each year. Sitting on the stage, watching the graduates walk by to receive their diplomas, he could not help feeling a sense of pride and gratification at the quality of these young people. One young man, who was graduating with honors, especially caught his eye, and he made a point to speak to him after the ceremony.

"Where will you be going to college in the fall, young man?" Bruce asked.

"I'm afraid I won't be going sir," he responded with a note of remorse and embarrassment. "We really can't afford it. And I need to get a job and help support my family."

The comment took Bruce back to the time when he was young and in a similar situation. But, in this day and age, he felt strongly that every young person, especially one with such promise, should have a chance at a better life. The boy's mother was standing beside him, and he asked her if they might come to his office in the morning. That evening, he made the decision to help support the fellow through his higher education, and the next day he shared his plan with an excited and grateful mother and son. That would be the first of many qualified young people whom he would support over the years with his own resources. And it was said that all of those students "made good."

Summer finally came and the end of school, and the Leslie children could think of nothing but the big trip they were about to take. Until, that is, the morning of their departure arrived. It was pitch dark when Bruce and Blossom got up and began attempting to rouse the children. Elizabeth and Ruth were reasonably cooperative, and Sam could be led around in his half-asleep state. But Frances was another matter. She had been out on a date the night before and had come in rather late. When she finally consented to get up, she slipped into the first thing she could find, which was the dress she had worn the night before. The other children were already out of the house and in the car, and she didn't have time to pack. And so, for the entire trip, she wore that same dress.

The two Fords, with which Bruce had begun his automotive experience, had long since been replaced by Buicks, which would be the family cars for the rest of his life. Their current Buick sedan comfortably seated three in the front seat and three in the back, which worked quite well for their family dynamics. Elizabeth and Frances, being only one year apart in age, were very close to each other, but did not include Ruth in most of their activities. As a result, Ruth had bonded with her brother, Sam, who was just one year younger than her. Although Ruth enjoyed her art and sewing, she also liked to play boys' games with Sam and later admitted that she was a bit of a tomboy. In any case, the pairing of the siblings (Elizabeth/Frances and Ruth/Sam) made for a good seating arrangement in the car, with the two sets alternating between the front and back seats. Bruce always drove, and Blossom sat in the back with whichever pair of her children were there at the time.

It was still dark as the family Buick pulled out of the gravel drive and onto Main Street, leaving the homestead in the rearview mirror. Frances and Sam were asleep before they were out of town, and the other two children soon followed suit. And so, as the family headed north on their big journey, Bruce and Blossom enjoyed the beauty of the sunrise alone and appreciated their quiet time together. Bruce had not seen Floy since she married Pope Batten and they had moved to South Dakota, though they had kept in close touch by mail over the years. Bruce was always good about writing, using his old typewriter and the "hunt and peck" method to turn out many letters. And yet it had been over thirty years since he had seen his sister, and he was very much looking forward to their visit.

Most of the roads in those days were single-lane and went through every little town, so travel was rather slow. By noon, they were just crossing the border into Kansas. Bruce found a grassy spot beside the road and pulled off for a mid-day break. Blossom had prepared a picnic lunch, which she took out from among all the luggage in the trunk. It was probably hunger that now had all the children wide awake. In any case, everyone was thankful to get out and stretch their legs and enjoy the meal. And then it was back on the road.

The drive through Kansas was quite a revelation for the children. They had no idea that any place could be so flat and devoid of trees. Mile after mile, they saw nothing but wheat fields and telephone poles. Their father jokingly said that the state tree of Kansas was the telephone pole. Sam thought that was a good joke, but the girls just rolled their eyes, and all four children agreed that this was not their favorite place. For Blossom and Bruce, however, it must have brought back some fond memories of a time when they were young and crossing the state from west to east on their honeymoon.

The sun was setting to their left as they approached the Nebraska state line. Their father found a roadside inn with a Vacancy sign and pulled in to inquire about accommodations and cost. Minutes later, he came back to the car to announce that this was where they would be spending the night. There was enough food left in the picnic basket for a reasonable supper, and the family sat on the porch of their cottage and enjoyed their evening meal, as the sun dropped beneath the vast midwestern prairieland. Elizabeth and Frances, however, did not seem to fully appreciate the tranquility of their situation. When they had first stepped inside the cottage, Frances saw a spider on the wall, which horrified her. And when they went back in after dinner, it only got worse.

"Daddy, there are spiders all over this place," Frances cried out.

"Well, they won't hurt you a bit," he reassured her in his calm tone. "When I was selling fruit trees, I used to sleep in barns, and there were spiders and a lot worse things."

That didn't seem to reassure Frances at all. She looked over at Elizabeth, who seemed equally horrified. They shook their heads and announced that they would sleep in the car. Their father told them to suit themselves. Ruth probably wished she could join them, but there wasn't room in the car for three. So she crawled in bed with her mother, pulled the sheet over her head, and tried to sleep.

Morning finally came, and the Leslie family was back on the road after finding breakfast at a local diner. It wasn't long before Sam began to wish he hadn't eaten so much. The constant swaying of the car and the warm day with no air conditioning was more than his little stomach could take. His father stopped the car and Blossom opened the door just in time for Sam to lose most of his breakfast. There were several more stops for such emergencies, which further slowed their progress, and by the time they finally crossed the border into South Dakota, Sam was fast asleep.

As they approached the Battens' home, they could see off to their left the silhouette of the Black Hills rising from the Great Plains of western South Dakota. Floy was in the front yard watching for them as they drove up the driveway. She could not hold back tears when she saw her brother for the first time in so many years, and Bruce wasn't doing much better with his emotions. He introduced his family, and then they all went into the lovely, spacious home where Pope and their children waited to meet the Leslies. The Battens owned a large department store, which had clothing sections for women and men, and the three sisters enjoyed browsing through the feminine apparel. It also had a grocery store, as well as a hardware section that was more to the taste of Sam and his father.

The Battens had a cabin on a river near the Black Hills, where everyone got to try their hand at trout fishing. There was also a gold mine nearby which they enjoyed touring. But the biggest attraction was a peak called Mount Rushmore into which the carving of four American presidents had been started just the year before.

On their last night, Bruce and Floy sat on the porch of her home and talked about their childhood, recalling the hard times after their father died and the day they rode the family mule together to take their teachers examination. They agreed that, despite all the challenges they had faced, life had been very good to them. They also talked about their lineage and how fortunate they were to have such a proud heritage. Then they held hands for a moment, closed their eyes, and said a prayer of thanks for all their blessings. And Bruce felt a gentle breeze caress his head.

The following morning, before the crack of dawn, the Leslies said goodbye to the Batten family, thanking them for such gracious hospitality. As they were preparing to get in the car, Floy and Pope gave each of them a lovely gift from their store as a memento of their time together. And then they were off. They each must have felt a bit of regret to be leaving the family that they had all come to love, but they were also looking forward to getting back to their home and their own lives. And undoubtedly the one who was most looking forward to that was Frances, who couldn't wait to change into a different dress.

And so life went on for the Leslie children. Elizabeth had a close friend, MaryMae, who was engaged to a fellow named Stanley. Elizabeth also had a boyfriend by the name of John Jared, and the four young people would often double date. Frances never lacked for suitors and seemed to always be going out with some young man. However, she was not only beautiful, kind, and sweet, but also quite prudent when it came to accepting male invitations. Her mother often sent her to the grocery store for needed items and, on one occasion, a young man who was working there asked her for a date.

Her polite but coy response was, "I'll have to ask my mother." And that was the end of that.

Ruth was at the awkward stage, somewhere between a little girl and a young lady. She still made time to play with Sam, once helping him build a two-story house out of boxes, for which she made curtains from old towels. But she was also beginning to have her own social life. A friend by the name of Helen Richards hosted a large party at the Hippodrome, to which Ruth was invited. She was rather proud when the local newspaper, the *Okmulgee Daily*, covered the event and listed all the attendees.

Sam also occasionally took notice of the local news and one day begged his mother to let him take an article to school for "show and tell." The year was 1931, and the article that caught Sam's eye was reporting the retirement of his father from the Okmulgee Board of Education after twenty-one years, sixteen of which he had served as president. Sam burst with pride when he read the front page headline, "Dr. Leslie Spent 21 Years Developing Schools." The lead paragraph stated, "If there is any one man in Okmulgee who may justly be credited with the lion's share of work in developing Okmulgee's school system, he is Dr. S. B. Leslie." When asked to weigh in, Superintendent Bruner was quoted to say, "It is a pleasure to work with such a man on the school board. Always prompt and faithful, quick to see the advantages of improvements. Dr. Leslie has made the way easier for the rapid advance of the Okmulgee schools." Those words captured the dedication that Bruce Leslie had given for over two decades to the growth of education in Okmulgee, and Sam and all his family were mighty proud.

◌֑ ֡◌

The Roaring Twenties came in the wake of World War I and brought a period of unprecedented economic prosperity in the United States and in many European nations, with large-scale expansion of the movie industry and ever-increasing use of automobiles, radio, and electrical appliances. The boom and the culture that came with it were experienced first in the large U.S. cities, but gradually worked their way into the smaller communities, including Okmulgee. Bruce did not think much of the flapper-style dresses and the dances that had his daughters so excited, but Blossom assured him that it was just a passing fancy. He would smile and shake his head and say that he hoped the fancy would pass quickly. What worried him far more was the way people seemed to be managing their finances. The stock market was robust, and many of his friends were investing heavily and reaping handsome profits. Bruce also invested but was careful to maintain a diversified portfolio and stay with well-established, reliable companies, such as Oklahoma-based Phillips Petroleum. Even then, it concerned him to have much of his wealth tied up in investments that could come and go all too easily. He looked at other investment vehicles and found real estate to be the most attractive.

He already owned one-fourth of the block on which they lived and had built three smaller houses on either side of the family home. One of them, right next door to the main house, had been occupied by Blossom's parents, and her brother, Charlie, continued to live there. The other two houses became rental properties, providing some additional income. But what Bruce believed to be the most promising real estate investment for the long-term was farmland. Much of the terrain around Okmulgee, being near the foothills of the Ozarks, was hilly, rocky, and heavily wooded. Interspersed among the rugged land, however, were flat areas which the early pioneers and the Native Americans before them had cleared and which now provided fertile soil for crops such as cotton, corn, and other vegetables. Most of these regions were only large enough to support small farms, but the favorable prices for produce and the transportation system that took them to distant markets made agriculture in the Twenties a profitable enterprise.

Bruce had become interested in the local farm scene from the day he returned to Okmulgee as a doctor. Since his practice frequently required house calls to farms in the surrounding countryside, he soon became familiar with the local farmland and agricultural methods. Often, after caring for his patient at one of the farms, he would sit down with the farmer and talk about their crops and the latest methods of farming. One aspect of crop growing that especially interested him was soil conservation. He listened carefully to the farmers he trusted most and read all he could about the importance of crop rotations and contour plowing, and that knowledge would prove vital in the years that lay ahead.

As his savings began to accumulate through hard work and frugal living, he decided in the early Twenties that it was time to start investing some of his money in the land around Okmulgee County. One day, when he had a break between patients in his office, he went next door to his friend, who was a real estate agent, and told him of his intent. The agent spread out a large map of the county, and they began looking at farm properties that were for sale. Bruce took notes and then began making special trips into the countryside to check out his options. He liked much of what he saw and soon returned to the agent to begin his acquisition of land. Over the years, he continued to acquire farmland in the region around Okmulgee, and his holdings eventually grew to over two thousand acres. (Most of that land, especially the mineral rights, is still in our family a century later.)

Some of the properties he acquired already had a house and other farm buildings on it, with tenant farmers who were leasing and farming the land. He assumed ownership of all the holdings on each farm and became the new landlord for the tenants. With other purchases, the land was undeveloped, and Bruce built homes and barns to lease to tenants. He created a friendly relationship with each of his tenant farmers and enjoyed driving out to visit them periodically to see how they were doing and to offer any help they might need. The only thing he required of them was adherence to good soil conservation practices—the contour plowing and planting, fertilizing, and anything else to preserve the soil. When the crops failed, he was always patient with the farmers and willing to give them another chance. However, a time was coming when his benevolence would be tested to the near limit.

⁘

As the decade of the Twenties was coming to an end, Bruce Leslie was well positioned financially. He was not making the same astounding profits that many of his friends were enjoying as the stock market continued to soar, but his modest investment portfolio, large land holdings, and busy medical practice gave him confidence that he was prepared for whatever the future might hold. Some of his friends felt that he was losing out by not taking advantage of the robust stock market. And indeed, by September of 1929, the Dow Jones had reached the remarkable peak of 381. But, three weeks later, Bruce picked up his morning paper to see that the Dow had fallen by nearly 13 percent, a day that would be remembered as "Black Thursday." Those friends who had so recently been sanguine about their investments now started to panic and began selling off their stocks. The same thing, of course, was happening all over the country, with the predictable results. By September 28, the Dow Jones had plummeted another 13 percent to 260. The following day would go down in history as "Black Tuesday," the day the Wall Street Stock Market crashed, triggering the Great Depression.

Dr. Leslie was not among those who immediately began selling off his stock portfolio. He listened to the experts who believed that the market would correct itself, and he followed their advice in hopes of riding out the storm. And, sure enough, although the Dow continued to fall over the next two months to a low of 198, it recovered to 294 by early 1930, and there was a renewed sense of optimism. But it was not to last.

Although the crash began in the United States, it soon spread worldwide. Congress attempted to shore up the economy by enacting tariffs, but other countries retaliated, exacerbating the problem and leading to a collapse in global trade. By 1932, the Dow dropped to a low of 41, and the following year, world trade fell to one-third of the prior four years. The world was truly in a depression.

Bruce Leslie felt the pain along with everyone else. He still had faith in his Republican Party, believing that Hoover would find a way out of the morass. When Franklin Roosevelt defeated Hoover in 1932, the doctor feared that the country would only fall into a worse financial condition. But he knew that the national situation was desperate, and his heart ached for all those who were suffering; he prayed that FDR's administration would find answers to lift the people out of their despair. Thanks to Bruce's careful approach to investment and his continued busy practice, his family was better off than most of those in Okmulgee. But even they had to be increasingly careful with their expenses. And, while his primary concern was for his own family, Bruce also felt an obligation to do what he could for others in their community. Many of them had lost everything and could no longer pay for their medical care. Bruce never denied care to those who could not pay, always accepting whatever they could afford, often in the form of a bartering of services or goods. Some had nothing to offer, and the doctor not only waived their charges, but would occasionally reach into his pocket and give his own money to a patient when he knew the family was going hungry.

And then there were his farms and the tenants who struggled to keep them going. In 1934, the Southwestern states were hit with yet another disaster: The Great Dustbowl. Many farmers had not paid attention to the call for soil conservation. Like the rest of the nation, they wanted quick returns on their investments, which often meant cutting corners on sound agricultural practices. When droughts came, the soil turned to dust, and then the winds swept across the barren fields, blowing away any hope of successful crops. Many Oklahoma farmers simply gave up and headed west. The eastern part of Oklahoma, which includes Okmulgee, being a hillier and more wooded part of the state, fared somewhat better than other regions, although the combination of depression and dustbowl had its effect there as well.

Bruce made frequent trips to the country to check on his farms and tenants, and what he found was often heartbreaking. Although most of the farmers had tried to follow his guidelines for soil conservation, crop failures were common during those desperate years. Families that had always lived on the edge of poverty now found themselves wondering where their next meal might come from. One Sunday after church, Bruce and his family drove out to one of his farms. They wondered if anyone was home, because there were no lights on in the little house and no sounds of life. But when they looked through the front door, which had been left open, they saw a family of seven sitting silently around a rough wood table. On the table was their Sunday dinner—one can of beans that they were all sharing.

Bruce required his tenants to pay only what they could, frequently accepting a basket of produce as payment. A bushel of potatoes or turnips could almost always be found on the back porch of the homestead. For those tenants who could not even afford that, he again took money out of his own pocket and did his best to see that no one went hungry during those desperate years.

Okmulgee fared better than many of the surrounding towns during the Depression because it was the county seat and received federal funds. In 1935, Roosevelt created the Works Progress Administration (WPA) as one of many measures to help mitigate the effect of the Depression. One of the WPA projects was to build a dam and spillway for Okmulgee Lake at the east end of Okmulgee State Park. An earthen dam, built in 1927, wasn't expected to last long, and the work project replaced it with a sturdy stone dam and spillway that today provides a beautiful lake and recreation area and is a major attraction of the county. Notwithstanding these enhancements and the federal support, however, the population of Okmulgee shrank during the Depression and never fully recovered.

Despite the exigencies of the Depression years, life went on for the Leslie family. Radios had become popular during the Twenties, but the Leslie family had yet to acquire one, much to the dismay of the three sisters, who loved the music of the day. By the early Thirties, however, the misfortunes of some, due to the Depression, were creating opportunities for others. Their father knew a man who had been forced to close his furniture store because of the hard times and was offering a radio at a bargain price. It may have been Bruce's desire to help the man, or to placate his daughters, or just to take advantage of a bargain. Whatever the reason, he bought the radio. It was actually a combination radio and phonograph in a beautiful wooden cabinet, with the phonograph on top and the radio in the bottom part. It was the first radio in their neighborhood, and Blossom occasionally invited her friends over for radio parties. The girls couldn't get enough of the music, especially songs like "Star Dust" and "Up a Lazy River." They swooned over Bing Crosby, who made his solo radio debut in 1931, and they saved their money to buy all the records they could.

In the evenings, the family would often sit together in the living room and listen to their favorite radio programs. They were especially fond of *The Jack Benny Show* and *The George Burns and Gracie Allen Show*, both of which debuted in 1932. Bruce's favorites, however, were *The Lone Ranger* and *Death Valley Days*, which he felt always had a good moral. And Sam loved listening to *Amos and Andy* and *The Aldrich Family*.

The family had a dog named Foxy, who also seemed to enjoy the radio and would sit with the family in the evening. Foxy, however, had a bad habit of howling, especially when out roaming the neighborhood, which made him rather unpopular with some of the neighbors. In fact, the poor dog had a bald spot on his back where a local apartment tenant had poured boiling water on him one night to stop the howling. The Leslies kept Foxy closer to home after that.

The 1930s was the decade of higher education for the Leslie children. It was also a time when they were old enough to take some trips on their own. Elizabeth and her friend MaryMae went to Colorado in 1934. MaryMae's fiancé, Stanley, accompanied them as their "chaperone." During that trip, the young ladies got their nerve up to do something rather daring—they wore slacks, which was quite a new thing for women at the time. The trip was a magical experience for the three young people, as they took in the majesty of the Rocky Mountains. For Elizabeth, it must have brought back memories of stories that her father had told the family about his years in Denver.

Upon her return from the Colorado trip, Elizabeth entered Oklahoma A&M in Stillwater, majoring in education. After two years, she transferred to Tahlequah Teachers College, from which she had intended to graduate. But she learned that a teacher was urgently needed in the little Oklahoma town of Shidler, and she called her father for his advice. Considering the difficult times in which they were still living, he felt that it was wise for her to apply for the position. He drove her and a friend to Shidler, so that both young ladies could apply. According to Elizabeth, her friend actually had better grades, but she had the advantage that her father was acquainted with the president of the school board there. In any case, Elizabeth got the position, and thus began her career in teaching.

Frances began her undergraduate education at Okmulgee Junior College as a cost-saving measure to minimize the financial impact on the family. After one year, she transferred to Oklahoma A&M. Throughout her college years, she continued to have many admiring suitors and never lacked for escorts to all of the school activities.

One of Frances's many virtues was the fact that "when she liked someone, she stuck with them." So, when one of her best friends enrolled at Tahlequah Teachers College, Frances decided to transfer there to be with her friend, as well as with Elizabeth. She apparently made that decision on her own and then told her father. She feared that he might be upset with her making the move on her own, but he agreed that it was a good plan, possibly because Tahlequah was less expensive. In the uncertain times of a depression and with four children to educate, it was imperative to be frugal whenever possible. Frances did well at Tahlequah, graduating with a degree in education. She then moved to Chickasha, Oklahoma, where she became a teacher like her sister Elizabeth.

When Ruth was a senior in high school, she received a letter from her Aunt Ollie in Santa Barbara, California. Her father's half-sister Ollie Brinks had been living there for several years with her husband, who was a grocer. The letter was an invitation for Ruth to visit them that summer before going off to college in the fall. The thought of traveling alone to such a faraway place—much farther away than she had ever been before—seemed quite daunting to her. It was even a bit frightening. But, at the same time, she found the idea very exciting. She discussed it with her parents, who also had mixed feelings about such an adventure for their youngest daughter. Her mother was reluctant, but her father saw it as a great opportunity—after all, he had been younger than Ruth when he had ventured off into Indian Territory by himself. In the end, they all agreed that it was too good to pass up.

And so, shortly after her graduation, Ruth boarded a train and headed out for "the trip of a lifetime." She couldn't get over how different California was from Oklahoma, especially when she stood for the first time on a sandy beach and looked out over the vast Pacific Ocean. Her aunt and uncle showed her a truly wonderful time, and she was a little sad when it was time to leave them. As a memento of her special trip, they gave her a set of exquisite little glass deer, which she treasured for the remainder of her life and are still in the family.

That fall, Ruth entered Okmulgee Junior College, as Frances had done. It was understood that this would only be for one year. During that year, she also expanded her social life. In the spring, she gave a bridge party for some friends and was delighted when it was covered in the local paper. She also continued her interest in art by joining the Palette and Brush Club. During her year in junior college, she applied to several universities and was thrilled to be accepted at the University of Arkansas. Her father was also pleased and proud, and he drove her to Fayetteville that fall. He helped her move into her dormitory and then said goodbye, leaving her all alone with no prospect of seeing any of her family before Thanksgiving. It didn't take long, however, for her to make friends, and her homesickness was partially assuaged when she was befriended by some young ladies from the Delta Delta Delta sorority who invited her to pledge. She called home for permission, but her father told her they couldn't afford it. When Elizabeth and Frances heard about this, they sent Ruth the money, and she became a Tri Delt for life, a path that her daughter and three granddaughters would one day follow.

Ruth enjoyed her year at Arkansas and especially the association with her Tri Delt sisters. But her goal had always been to study art, and she learned from her art instructor at the university that one of the best places for that was the Kansas City Art Institute. She called home to discuss it with her father, who had long since recognized his daughter's artistic talent, and he agreed that this was a reasonable path for her. She applied and, much to her surprise and delight, was accepted for the fall semester. And so father and daughter were soon on the road together once again, this time traveling to Kansas City.

The four Leslie children all loved and idolized their father. But for Sam the feeling went even deeper. He coveted the approval of his father and yearned to be as much like him as possible. More than any of his sisters, he took every opportunity he could to go on house calls with his father, and eventually he decided that he wanted to follow in his father's footsteps and become a physician. After the first two years at Okmulgee Junior College, he transferred to Northeastern State Teachers College at Tahlequah, where he completed his requirements for pre-med and then matriculated at the University of Oklahoma School of Medicine.

Bruce and Blossom were understandably proud that all their children had attended college and were well on their way to having fulfilling and productive lives. It had not been easy, especially during the Depression, and sacrifices were made by everyone in the family.

Even Uncle Charlie, who had been able to keep his job as a machinist, saved every penny he could and gave it to his nieces and nephew to help with their higher education. Bruce was grateful for that and thankful for the good fortune that had helped his family through the Depression, and he never failed to remember the source of their blessings or to thank God many times each day for the good health and success of their children and for the relative prosperity of his family. And yet he saw changes occurring in far-off places that gave him grave concern about the future for his family, the country, and the world.

For several years now, Bruce had been following the news out of Europe, which he found to be increasingly disturbing. As far back as 1921, he had read about Hitler, who had become leader of a minor political party in Germany. At the time, it didn't look like it would amount to much, especially three years later when Hitler was tried for treason in a failed coup and sentenced to five years of labor. Bruce thought he sounded mentally unstable and hoped that would be the end of him. But, just nine months after his imprisonment, the man was freed, and the news that followed became progressively alarming.

The year after his release from prison, Hitler resurrected the Nazi Party and started his inexorable rise to power. By 1933, the Nazis were gaining a large number of seats in the Reichstag, and President Hindenburg appointed Hitler to the position of Reich Chancellor. Within days of his appointment, disconcerting reports began to appear in the news: book burnings, banning of all other parties, even purging in his own Nazi party. Most concerning were the increasing restrictions on persons of the Jewish faith. And then, in 1934, Hitler merged the positions of president and chancellor and declared himself the "leader," which in German is the Führer. And Bruce Leslie could only wonder and worry about what would come next.

CHAPTER 12

Weddings and War

O N A COOL FALL AFTERNOON IN 1936, Dr. Leslie saw the last patient in his office and then drove out into the country to make one house call before going home. His drive that day took him north of town past Okmulgee Lake where men were still working on the stone dam and spillway, as part of the WPA program. The patient he was going to see was especially worrisome. She had diabetes, which was not particularly common in those days, since people didn't tend to live long with it. Insulin had only been isolated in the previous decade, and physicians were just recently understanding how to use it for their patients. Bruce Leslie had started his patient on it a couple of months earlier and worried about the dosage he had prescribed. Either too much or too little could put her into a life-threatening diabetic coma, and that is what dominated the doctor's thoughts as he followed the winding, narrow, tree-lined road that eventually brought him to her house.

As he walked into their home, with his black leather bag in one hand, he was relieved to find his patient in the kitchen preparing her family's dinner. She admitted that there were times she felt shaky, but the dietary schedule and insulin regimen that he had prescribed seemed to be working. He checked her vital signs and was pleased (and greatly relieved) to find that they were stable. They reviewed her daily schedule, trying to balance her diet and activity, and Bruce was satisfied that she was doing everything properly. He then asked her and her husband how they were doing and got the usual glum picture of a family barely able to get by, especially now with the added cost of her insulin. What they didn't know was that their doctor was only charging them a fraction of the cost of the medicine and was covering the rest out of his own pocket. He also told them not to worry about their medical bill until they were in a better position to pay it. They gave him a small basket of turnips and, although he was reluctant to accept even that, he did so with a show of sincere gratitude, which he felt was important to preserve their self-respect.

And so, with a feeling of relief for his patient, he said his farewells and headed home. By now, it was starting to get dark, and he turned on his headlights, since the winding roads and narrow shoulders could be difficult to follow at this time of day. There were no other cars on the road that evening, and his thoughts shifted from his patient to his own safety. The Depression was still plaguing the nation and the world, and some people had turned to crime as the only way they knew to provide food for themselves and their families. The increase in crime created yet another layer of fear during those dark times. Everyone had to be especially vigilant, and Bruce was intently aware of this as he drove slowly down the dark road.

As he approached an especially tight hairpin turn, he slowed down even more and, when he came around the curve, a man was right in front of him at the edge of the road, illuminated by the headlights. He thought the person looked suspicious and was just beginning to speed up, when the man jumped on his running board and grabbed the door handle.

Bruce had heard that this was how criminals were stealing cars and robbing the owners, and he knew there was only one way to avoid becoming one of those victims. He floor-boarded his car and, with tires screeching, cut sharply into the oncoming lane, which fortunately was empty. Going as fast as his Buick could muster, he kept weaving back and forth between the two lanes, as his attacker struggled desperately to hold on. Finally, with one especially violent cut, the man could hold on no longer and fell off onto the grassy shoulder.

As Bruce drove on, he wondered if the man was hurt and might need his care. But, when he looked in his rearview mirror, he saw him standing up and shaking his fist at the speeding car. He felt, therefore, that he was justified in going on, and it was only then that he noticed his own hands were shaking uncontrollably. As he continued driving home slowly and very cautiously, he said a prayer of sincere gratitude for having been spared a robbery or possibly worse, and he also said a prayer for his assailant.

When he arrived home that evening, he was still shaking and greatly disturbed, but he elected not to tell Blossom about the incident, since he didn't want her to worry. The house seemed nearly empty in those days with all three girls away at school or working. Sam was still living at home, finishing his last year at Okmulgee Junior College before going to Northeastern to complete his studies in pre-med. His father had been pleased when Sam had announced his intentions to pursue a career in medicine. There had not been a very close father-son relationship in Sam's youth, because his father was always so busy with his medical practice, his civic and church responsibilities, and his business dealings. But now they both seemed to enjoy the interaction that their common interest in medicine offered. Sam had been reading about diabetes and was especially interested to hear about the patient that his father had just visited.

As the two men were chatting in the living room, Blossom came in to announce that a letter had arrived earlier in the day from Elizabeth. It contained some rather exciting news about a certain young man she had met. She was teaching at Hay Creek School in Webb City, which is near Shidler, and had been invited to take the lead role in their faculty play. Elizabeth was shy by nature, and her only prior experience in performing before an audience had been singing with her school's Glee Club. But she had risen to the occasion and, by all accounts, had been a hit. At that time, she only weighed ninety-eight pounds and was very slender. For her performance, she wore a dress she had borrowed from Ruth. It was a slinky, low-cut, purple velvet dress, in which she apparently caught the attention of all the young men in the audience. But there was one man that evening who was especially taken by her. His name was Harold Hunsaker.

Harold had grown up in Kansas in the town of Port Lease, near El Dorado. In the midst of the Depression, his father broke his arm at work and was laid off, which meant that Harold had to find a job and do what he could to help support his family. His sister, Opal, and her husband, Elgin Cooper, had already moved to Shidler, where Elgin was employed by Phillips Petroleum Company. With the help of his brother-in-law, Harold was also able to get a job with Phillips and was already living in Webb City when Elizabeth came there for her teaching position.

After seeing Elizabeth in the school play, Harold could not get her out of his mind but didn't know how to go about meeting her. Then one day, he had gone to the post office, and there she was. She had come in to get her mail. He hoped to catch her eye, but she went straight to her mailbox, without looking left or right, got her mail, and departed. He returned to the post office at the same time the next day in hopes of seeing her again and, sure enough, there she was, but still focused on her mission. This scenario played out several more times over the following days, and Harold was just about to give up hope, when he heard about an Elks dance in nearby Ponca City.

He had hoped that Elizabeth might be at the dance, and he hadn't been there long before he saw her walk in. But his heart sank when he realized that she had come with another man, a fellow by the name of Jack Baker. She was double-dating with her friends MaryMae and Stanley. In those days it was considered improper to strike up a conversation with a stranger, so Harold enlisted the help of a friend, Russell Davidson, who happened to know Elizabeth. While she was dancing with Jack, Russell cut in and proceeded to tell her about this friend of his. When the dance was over, Russell introduced Elizabeth to Harold, and it didn't take long after that for the romance to begin.

This is the story, in part, that Blossom related to Bruce and Sam from the letter that they had just received from Elizabeth. Her daughter made it clear that she and Harold were in love and that matrimony was on the horizon. However, both young people felt that they had reasons to delay the wedding. Harold was trying to help his parents move closer to where he was living. Elizabeth would not be allowed to continue teaching if she was married, and she needed the money to buy furniture for their future home. And so it was agreed that they would have an extended engagement of two years before their wedding.

The big day, June 7, 1937, finally came. The wedding, held in the Leslie home, was a modest affair, attended only by family members. Elizabeth wore a pink dress and hat, her favorite color, and carried a bouquet of pink roses. Frances was her maid of honor, and Ruth, just back from Arkansas, was the bridesmaid. A friend of Harold was scheduled to serve as best man, but they learned at the last minute that he couldn't make it, and Sam filled in for him. As the wedding march played, Elizabeth came down the oak stairs on her father's arm. One of the steps had a tendency to squeak, and when daughter and father reached it, Frances thought the sound was that of her mother or grandmother McKeage crying. When she mentioned it later, both women denied it, but it made for a good family laugh. In any case, it was said to be a lovely wedding, although there is no photographic documentation, since no one thought to take pictures. But the young couple undoubtedly stored enough memories of that day to last a lifetime.

In the fall of the same year, Ruth entered the Kansas City Art Institute and would soon experience her own romantic adventures. The Institute offered classes in a wide range of artistic endeavors. She enjoyed studying perspective, sketching with pencil, charcoal, and pen and ink, and painting in watercolor and other media. But possibly her favorite course, which combined her passion for art and sewing, was fashion design. In the spring, she entered a contest, along with thirty-two of her fellow students, to design, fabricate, and model an ensemble. Hers was a tailored suit, which had a little twist to it: the suit included an accessory which she flipped over to become a purse as she stood on the stage. It was enough to win first prize of $25.

Although Kansas City had been a cultural shock at first after Okmulgee and even Fayetteville, Ruth soon found herself loving all the opportunities that it had to offer. She made a small circle of friends, and they enjoyed going to art galleries, museums, and parks, most of which offered free admission. She lived in a boardinghouse with other young women, and that turned out to be the most significant of all her experiences in Kansas City. For their evening meal, the women sat around a large dining room table and were served by young men who were students at the various schools in the city. Ruth began to notice that one of them seemed to be paying special attention to her. His name, she learned, was Bishop Shields.

Bishop had grown up in Enid, Oklahoma, with his brother, Herb, and his sister, Maurine. His father was a dentist and, like Sam Leslie, Bishop had chosen to follow in his father's footsteps. He earned his bachelor's degree at Phillips University in Enid, where the president was Eugene Briggs, the same man Bruce Leslie had initially brought to Oklahoma as an administrator in the Okmulgee school system. Bishop then matriculated at the Kansas City School of Dentistry. In order to help pay for his room and board, he took a part-time job as a server, busboy, and dishwasher in Ruth's boardinghouse.

As would be expected, each of the young men studied the ladies around the table and decided which ones they found to be most appealing. Bishop Shields was no exception, and his eyes were soon for only one person: Miss Ruth Leslie. But the problem was how to meet her. After several weeks of seeing her at the evening meals, Bishop finally worked up his nerve to speak to Ruth.

"Would you care for more potatoes, Miss Leslie?"

Ruth looked up, and their eyes met for the first time.

"No, thank you," she replied, "but they were very good."

Bishop blushed, nodded, and moved on. *They were very good,* she had said. Those simple words gave him hope. Even though he had only served the potatoes, she liked something about him. From then on, he routinely asked her if she cared for seconds. The only thing he learned from that was that she didn't eat much. But it was an opening, and gradually they began to have brief conversations after dinner. He knew of her interest in art and finally worked up the courage to ask her if she would like to attend a new exhibit with him. She accepted, it went well, and another romance in the Leslie family began. As the courtship advanced, they were both pleased to discover that they came from similar backgrounds and had similar values and interests. Finally, Bishop popped the big question and couldn't wait to call his family to tell them that she had accepted.

"She's a swell gal," he began. "Mom, you're going to love her because she sews. Maurine, you'll love her because she's a Tri Delt. And Dad, you're going to love her because she's a real looker."

Bishop graduated from dental school that spring and started his dental practice in the tiny Oklahoma town of Hydro. Ruth elected not to return to the Art Institute in the fall and stayed home to prepare for the wedding. And then, on June 3, 1939, Bruce and Blossom Leslie celebrated the second wedding of one of their children.

This time the wedding was held in the First Methodist Church of Okmulgee. According to the local society page, Ruth wore a bouffant white lace and net dress over a white satin slip. Her bouquet was of gladiola bells, stephanotis, and lilies-of-the-valley. Frances was the maid of honor, and Bishop's sister, Maurine, was one of four bridesmaids. Bishop's brother, Herb, was the best man, and Sam Leslie and Maurine's fiancé, Jack Wilson, were two of the four ushers. Elizabeth was consumed with being a new mother for their one-year-old daughter, Frances Ann, but was able to assist in serving at the reception.

And so, for the second time, Dr. S. B. Leslie extended his arm to escort a daughter to the altar. As they walked slowly down the aisle, to the organ strains of Lohengrin's *Bridal Chorus*, he looked out at the host of well-wishers. There were the Kennedys, the Trents, and the McIntoshes. A number of his patients had come, along with medical colleagues and people he had worked with on the school board and in his church. And one can only guess what thoughts were going through his mind at that moment: possibly about the first time he came to Okmulgee, when he was younger than the woman on his arm; or when he returned, years later, with a degree in medicine; or when he brought his young bride to their new home; or when she gave birth to each of their four children. Whatever he was thinking, it is quite certain that he was offering a silent prayer of thanks for all his blessings.

But it is also likely that he was troubled about the future for his daughter and all his family as they faced a world of many uncertainties. Just the year before, Hitler had seized control of the German Army, and one month later Nazi Germany invaded and annexed Austria. All the world was now holding its collective breath to see what would happen next. With their children and in-laws just starting out in adult life, Dr. Leslie could not help but worry about what the future held for them.

Three months after Ruth's wedding, her father picked up the morning paper and read the headlines that he had hoped to never see. The Nazi Army had invaded Poland, and Great Britain had declared war on Germany. World War II had begun. FDR declared neutrality for the United States, but Bruce feared it would only be a matter of time before all the world would be drawn into the conflict. He shuddered to think what this would mean for his children's generation.

When their daughter, Frances Ann, was born on November 29, 1938, Harold and Elizabeth were living in company housing on a section of oil fields in northeastern Oklahoma known as Burbank Field. Their home was in an area called Vinnage Camp, which was near the town of Fairfax. The town had a hospital, which proved to be a blessing, since Elizabeth had gone into shock after the delivery and come close to dying. Shortly thereafter, they moved to Hyatt Camp, which Elizabeth disliked because it was more remote from a town of any size and a hospital. And her concern would soon be justified following the arrival of their second child.

On June 6, 1940, Elizabeth gave birth to their son, Harold, who would be called Hal. When he was six months old, Hal contracted pneumonia and might have died had they not been able to rush him to the nearest doctor. He was treated with sulfa, and the outcome was good, but Elizabeth continued to worry about their lack of proximity to medical care. Before long, it was Francie Ann who would justify her mother's concern when she fell and cut her wrist on a dirty tin can. Again, it was a rush to the closest doctor. A neighbor drove them, while Elizabeth keep pressure on her daughter's wrist so she wouldn't bleed to death. Again, the outcome was good, but Elizabeth was understandably relieved when the family moved to a large, comfortable home near Shidler, which remained the family homestead for the remainder of her life.

Of course, everyone in the Leslie family continued to follow world events with great trepidation. And it wasn't looking good. In the spring of 1940, Germany invaded France, which surrendered within two months. Several other European countries also fell to the Nazis, and the Allied forces were in retreat by late May. More than 300,000 troops, trapped on a beach near Dunkirk in the north of France, were saved when England rallied with some 800 civilian vessels. At about the same time, Winston Churchill was elected Prime Minister, and three months later the German Luftwaffe began a relentless bombing of London and other British cities. America remained neutral, but was ramping up production of ships, planes, and other necessities of war and was enlisting thousands of young men who were stirred by patriotism or by the continued ravages of the Depression.

Frances Leslie was still teaching in Chickasha, about 100 miles southwest of Okmulgee. She had now been the maid of honor for both of her sisters but seemed to have no prospects of her own. This did not appear to concern her, however, nor did it concern anyone who knew her well, as she had a line of young men who longed for her heart. She had reddish hair, a soft, sweet face, a perpetual twinkle in her eye, and a zest for life. She never lacked for suitors, but the right man had simply not yet come along. A USO had been established at a nearby training center in Norman, Oklahoma, and Frances volunteered to work there, which must have been a comfort to the young recruits who were already feeling homesick. She enjoyed doing what she could to make their lives a little more pleasant, but worried greatly about what the future held for them.

Meanwhile, back in Okmulgee, Dr. Leslie continued his hectic schedule. He was still supporting the Methodist Church and was also helping other churches, including a small country church a few miles outside of town. In addition to having served on the school board for many years and holding leadership roles in a variety of local and state medical groups, he had joined the local Masonic Order Lodge #199 and was serving on the Building and Loans board of his bank and on the municipal cemetery board. For several years, he was an alternate on the State Board of Medical Examiners, which issues licenses to practice medicine in the state. And then, beginning in 1940, he was appointed by two Oklahoma governors to serve two four-year active terms on the board. He did all this while maintaining a busy medical practice and managing his business interests. But, like everyone else, his mind was constantly occupied with the ominous state of world affairs.

After their wedding and a short honeymoon, Ruth joined Bishop in Hydro, Oklahoma. But the small town and hard times simply could not support a dentist, so the young couple moved to Lawton, Oklahoma, where Bishop served as a dentist for the National Youth Agency (NYA). They lived in a dormitory on the campus of Cameron

College, and it was there that Ruth informed Bishop that, come spring, they would be having their first child. Bishop had enlisted in the National Guard, and his division, the 45th, also known as the Thunderbirds, was activated in late 1940. He was ordered to report to Abilene, Texas, to begin basic training.

Ruth returned to Okmulgee to live with her folks while Bishop was in Abilene, and it was there, on April 22, 1941, that she gave birth to their first child (the author). They named him Milton Brewster, but later changed it to Bruce because the longer name was apparently too hard for the young child to spell. Upon learning of his son's arrival, Bishop jumped in his old car and headed for Okmulgee. Along the way, one of the headlights fell off, but he was not about to let that slow him down. He just tossed the headlight in the back seat and kept going.

So 1941 got off to a good start for the Shields family, but the year would end tragically for everyone. On a chilly Sunday morning in early December, Bishop and Ruth, who were now reunited in Abilene, took their infant son to church on the base. Harold and Elizabeth went to their church in Shidler with their two young children, while Frances worshiped in Chickasha. Bruce and Blossom Leslie, as always, attended the First Methodist Church in Okmulgee. Driving home, Bruce turned on the car radio to catch the news. As they listened to the breaking report, he slowed the car and pulled over to the curb. He looked over at Blossom and took her hand, as tears welled up in her eyes. The day was December 7, and they had just learned of the bombing of Pearl Harbor. They knew what this meant for the young men in their family and for so many young men and women across the country. They closed their eyes and said a prayer.

The Hunsaker family was blessed that Harold was not called into military service. Being thirty-two years of age with a wife and two children and working in the petroleum industry, which was critical to the war effort, he was exempted. Sam Leslie was less fortunate. He was just finishing medical school at the University of Oklahoma, and virtually all graduates were being drafted. His assignment was with the Army and, after a brief training program, his division was sent to England and told that they would eventually be going to Paris. Bishop's 45th Division had further training in Upstate New York and Massachusetts and was then deployed to Europe. Ruth and her infant son were able to join him for part of his time in the Northeast and then returned to Okmulgee to wait out the war.

Okmulgee, like every other town in the country, focused all its resources on the war effort. The Creek Council House became the Red Cross headquarters, where clothing was made and gathered by volunteers. People of all ages went about town collecting scrap metal, which was vitally needed. In 1943, the federal government built the Glennan Military Hospital in Okmulgee. It was first used to care for injured American servicemen, but later it took in German POWs who were in prison camps around the state. Some of those prisoners, when they had sufficiently recovered, were hired to work on farms around the county. Rationing became a way of life. In 1942, it was primarily sugar and gasoline, and by 1943 there was general food rationing, as everyone felt the effects of war.

The war years were particularly hard on Bruce and Blossom. On top of his busy medical practice and civic duties and her never-ending household responsibilities, they both volunteered wherever they could for the war effort. But what made it especially hard was their strong aversion to war in general and their overwhelming sense of anguish for all the young lives that were cut short. And yet, Dr. Leslie had to admit that some good did seem to come indirectly from the war. In his case, it was the development of new medicines. Throughout his career as a physician, the patients who worried him the most were those with infectious diseases. He had watched too many of them die for lack of effective antimicrobials. Although penicillin had been discovered in 1928 by the British scientist Alexander Fleming, it took more than a decade to understand how to use it in patients. The first human injection was not given until 1941 in Oxford, England, and even then, there was the problem of how to produce it in sufficient quantities. The pharmaceutical companies in Great Britain were too busy with wartime efforts to study the issue, so it fell to the American drug industry. The first use of penicillin in the United States was a case at Yale University in 1942, and by 1944 the drug was generally available. The introduction of antibiotics may have been the greatest advance in medical science during the twentieth century and was a great relief for Dr. Leslie and for all physicians.

The Leslie family, like families the world over, followed the news of the war intently on their radio. Ruth knew only that her husband's division was somewhere in western Europe. Then, in late January of 1944, she learned that the 45th Division was part of the invasion of Italy at the Anzio Beachhead. It was said to be one of the most bitterly contested pieces of land in the war, and Ruth could only pray that Bishop had survived. Six months later, the Allied forces landed on Omaha Beach in Normandy, launching D-Day. Sam Leslie had been scheduled to go to Paris after D-Day, but his division did not deploy before the war in Europe ended on May 8, 1945. He was then assigned to a troop ship in the Pacific but was again fortunate when the Japanese surrendered in August of that year.

Now the war was over. Sam came home safely, finally able to begin his practice of general medicine. Bishop returned to his wife and four-year-old son and they prepared to start their life in Enid. Bishop's brother, Herb, and his brother-in-law, Jack Wilson, both of whom had served overseas in the Army, also came back safely. So the Leslies and all their extended family had much to be thankful for, and they did not fail to recognize the source of their blessings and to offer profound thanks.

CHAPTER 13

The Grands

ON A WARM MORNING IN EARLY AUGUST, S. B. slipped quietly from his side of the bed and stretched his lanky frame. His hair was now silver and thinning—the way his grandchildren would always remember him—but he was still slender and stood tall and straight except for the slight familial stoop of his shoulders. He stepped gingerly into the hall, trying to avoid stepping on the floorboards that had long since begun to squeak.

The old family home was still sturdy, but the neighborhood that surrounded it had deteriorated over the years. When Bruce had built the house more than forty years earlier, it was the only structure on the block and was in a respectable location within convenient walking distance of his office downtown. With the passage of the decades, however, many changes had occurred in the neighborhood that created a less than ideal environment. The Leslie home faced East Third Street, and smaller houses had long since filled up the neighborhood on that end of the block and were now looking rather tired. One positive feature was a small grocery store called Gilstrap's directly across East Third from the Leslie home, which was convenient for Blossom.

The town had grown out to encompass the other end of the block, and the municipal fire station had been built just across the gravel drive that led up to the Leslie home. Adjacent to the fire station and occupying the remainder of the block on the town side were several large industrial buildings. Across Main Street from the family home was a cotton gin, and the creek that ran by it was now polluted and commonly referred to as Greasy Creek.

Many townspeople wondered why such a prominent doctor and community leader didn't move to one of the newer residential parts of town. He could have easily afforded a better home, but his frugality and possibly the memories the old house held for him were such that he didn't even consider moving. Besides, there were other things in the life of Dr. Leslie that were far more important to him.

The house was nearly empty on that August morning. The only occupants, aside from himself and Blossom, were my mother and me. The war in Europe was coming to a close, and my father would soon be coming home to start our new life. But Sam's division had received orders to transfer to the Pacific theater, where the war with Japan still raged. This weighed heavily on Bruce Leslie, as he walked slowly down the oak stairs and entered the kitchen. As he had done every morning for nearly half a century, he opened his Bible, read his scripture for the day, and said his prayers, with a special, fervent petition for his son. Then, after preparing his breakfast and pouring his coffee, he sat down to read the morning paper. And the headlines that jumped out at him that morning nearly took his breath away.

Across the top of the front page in large, bold letters was the announcement that the United States had dropped a terrible bomb—an atomic bomb—on a city in Japan. The devastation was apparently beyond imagination, and Bruce's first thought was for all the innocent people who would suffer and die. But then he realized that such a weapon would surely force Japan to surrender and bring the war to an end. And that meant that Sam would be coming home. So he again closed his eyes and bowed his head and offered a prayer of thanksgiving for his son's safety and also a petition for all those afflicted in Japan.

Sam Leslie did indeed return home safely from the war, and there was rejoicing on East Third Street. But, for Bruce Leslie at least, the joy was not to last long. Sam felt that he had lost time and must move on with his medical career. His father was hoping that he would set up practice in Okmulgee and asked his son about it.

"Well, sir," Sam began hesitantly. "I feel like I need help in re-entering civilian medicine, and there is a position at a government hospital in Clinton where they primarily treat TB patients. I think that might give me some valuable experience before I decide on my private practice."

His father was silent and pensive for a moment. It seemed that there was a touch of sadness in his eyes. He was now seventy-one years old, still practicing full-time, and looking forward to the day when his son might join him in his practice. Time was running out for the realization of such an opportunity, and yet he understood Sam's reasoning and quietly nodded his approval.

Two years at the hospital in Clinton, Oklahoma, flew by quickly for Sam. He enjoyed the work and felt it was profitable in his continuing medical education. But one experience during those years would forever stand alone in his memory. He was on duty at the hospital when an emergency call came in from the town of Woodward, Oklahoma. They had been hit by a tornado and were requesting that several ambulances and doctors and nurses be sent as soon as possible. Sam and his partner on duty were in the doctor's lounge when the call came. Sam put his hand over the phone to relay the information to his partner. The medical staff at Woodward had gained a reputation of asking for help when it was not always necessary. The two young doctors had gotten a bit tired of it, and they rolled their eyes and shook their heads, thinking this was most likely just another false alarm. But, when he returned to the phone, Sam very politely said, "Yes, of course, we will be there as quickly as we can."

It was dark by the time they got on the road, and the weather was terrible. As two ambulances sped down the highway toward Woodward, one hit a slick patch and spun out of control. It crashed into a tree beside the road, injuring the driver, doctor, and nurse. Fortunately, no one was killed, but it added to the irritation of Sam and his partner, who were in the other ambulance. They thought this had better be a legitimate call for the price they were paying. But when they arrived, what they saw was beyond anything they could have imagined.

During the war, Sam had witnessed the massive destruction of towns in England from the relentless bombing by Nazi Germany and felt certain that he would never again see anything like it in his lifetime. And yet, as they drove into Woodward, he realized that he was seeing destruction at an entirely new level. Entire swaths of the town were simply gone. Where homes had once stood, there were now only foundations. Sam and his team worked through the night treating the injured, and the sun was well up before they were able to take a break and eventually return to their own hospital. For the rest of his life, Sam Leslie would never forget the Woodward Tornado of 1947.

Three months later, S. B. received a letter at his office. It was from Sam, and that alone lifted the older doctor's spirits. The last time the two had corresponded was just after the tornado, and he had continued to wonder about their future together. He still longed for the day when his son might join his practice, and the opening sentences of the letter gave him renewed hope. Sam had decided to leave Clinton and return to Okmulgee to set up practice. Bruce felt almost giddy to think that his dream could be coming true. He had always regretted not having a closer relationship with Sam when he was growing up, and he had rejoiced the day his son announced that he had decided to follow in his father's footsteps and become a doctor. That common interest seemed to bring the two Leslie men closer together, and he prayed that Sam would one day accept his offer to join his practice. But, as he continued reading the letter, he felt all that hope draining from him.

Sam explained that he and an old friend, Donald McCauley, had decided to set up practice together in a modern office building a few blocks from the town square. Bruce read the letter several times and then let it fall on his lap. He sat quietly, looking out the window of his now antiquated office. Was that why Sam didn't want to join him? Because his facilities were no longer state-of-the-art? Or was he ashamed that his father did not have a traditional medical degree? Despite his decades of success as a respected physician in the community and among his medical peers statewide, it had always bothered Bruce that his degree was as a Doctor of Homeopathy. As he continued to ponder his son's decision, he had to admit that it was understandable for him to want to go into partnership with a young friend and to be in a modern office. So he took a deep breath and resigned himself to the fact of the matter. But he noticed that there was a tear in his eye.

During the war, Frances had continued to teach school in Chickasha. She still had her ardent suitors, although the number had dwindled as many young men were off serving their country. She had also continued to work at the nearby USO and met many men there, most of whom were either married or had sweethearts. She was now in her early thirties and beginning to wonder if she had passed up too many marriage prospects along the way and if the right man would ever come along.

On most weekends, she would come home to her family in Okmulgee. If she was concerned about her future, it never showed in her perpetual effervescent spirit. During the time that my mother and I were living in Okmulgee, Aunt Frances was like a second mother to me, and I suspect that my mother was grateful to have a little relief in caring for me when her sister was home. In the summer of 1945, as the war was coming to a close, Frances spent more of her time at the family home. That turned out to be quite propitious. During the summer, her father came down with the flu, and for the first time since his fateful illness in Denver he found himself confined to his bed. Frances stayed by his side, doing whatever she could to make him comfortable. One day, when he was feeling better but still unable to get out of bed, he asked her to go downtown to pay their gas bill. And that simple request would change her life.

As Frances walked into the Oklahoma Natural Gas building, she noticed a handsome man, about her age, sitting behind a desk with a sign that indicated he was the office manager. She was embarrassed to find herself staring at him, but then realized that he was also looking at her. Frances felt that she knew him but couldn't remember where they might have met. She proceeded to the counter, paid the bill, and turned to leave. But the man looked up at her again, and she couldn't resist looking toward him. At that point, they both laughed a bit self-consciously, and Frances broke the ice.

"Do I know you?" she asked.

"It's possible," he replied. "My name is Glen Echols."

And then it all came flooding back to her. When she had been a sophomore at Oklahoma A&M, living in Thatcher Hall, she dated a fellow who had a roommate named Glen. One evening, her boyfriend invited her to his room for dinner, and Glen prepared the meal. She remembered thinking that he was very nice, but he never asked her for a date, and she had pretty much forgotten about him. But here he was, right in front of her, after all those years.

Glen Echols was born in Seminole, Oklahoma, and grew up in nearby Quinton. He loved the out-of-doors and enjoyed camping, fishing, and scouting. When he grew to manhood, he continued his interest in Boy Scouts and became a Scout leader. He was a "man's man" with rugged good looks and a quiet but friendly personality. He lost both of his parents at a young age and married in his early twenties. In 1936, the couple had a child, whom they named Tom Ed. The marriage didn't work out, but father and son stayed together, and the mother drifted out of the picture. So now, in his early thirties, Glen was a single father raising his young son.

Frances and Glen spent the next several minutes talking about their common past and where life had taken them since those college days. Finally, she told him that she needed to return home to take care of her father. He watched her walk out of the ONG building and the next day he called her for a date. Thus began the third romance among the Leslie sisters. One of my earliest memories as a four-year-old is being taken with them on some of their dates, particularly to Okmulgee Lake. All I can really recall is their kindness to me and a feeling of warmth and happiness in their midst.

Glen eventually proposed to Frances, and wedding plans were again a topic of discussion in the Leslie household. But Frances insisted that she did not want a big wedding. She said that she had experienced a lovely home wedding and a gorgeous church wedding with her two sisters and that she desired neither. All she wanted was to be married by the preacher in their Methodist church, with her mother as her maid of honor and her father by her side and Glen with his best man. Her mother tried to talk her out of it, but Frances was adamant, and she got her way. For her wedding present, she asked her parents to buy her a pearl gray suit, which she wore in the wedding and continued to wear for many years thereafter. She had much of her father's frugality.

Not long after their wedding, Glen received a promotion and was transferred to Sapulpa, which is about thirty miles from Okmulgee. There they bought a small, comfortable house on a pleasant, tree-lined street and the three of them settled in to begin their new life. They hadn't been there long before Frances informed Glen that their family would soon grow to four. On August 31, 1948, she gave birth to their second son, whom they named Samuel Glenn and called Sam. With 12 years difference in their ages, young Sam looked up to his big brother Tom Ed, and the three men of the Echols family bonded in their love for scouting and the outdoor life, while Frances felt content and blessed in the comfort and love of her little family. The news of their fifth grandchild was greeted with great joy in Okmulgee by Bruce and Blossom (and it partially assuaged Bruce's disappointment when, two months after Sam's birth, Harry Truman upset Thomas Dewey in the presidential election).

As the country entered the post-war era in 1946, Elizabeth and Harold Hunsaker and their two children were also enjoying the peace and contentment of a close, loving family. Their home near Shidler was situated in the country on oil field property where Harold worked. When my family visited them in later years, I remember being rather envious of my cousin Hal, as I witnessed all the amenities that country living had to offer, especially the horse that Hal owned. Back in Okmulgee, our grandparents naturally wanted to see their grandchildren as often as possible, but an unfortunate event associated with the marriage of Elizabeth and Harold put a temporary strain on visits with the Hunsakers.

Blossom's mother, Nettie McKeage, had still been living in the house next door when Elizabeth announced her intention to marry Harold. While Elizabeth's parents were supportive of the marriage, her Grandmother McKeage told her that she would "never forgive her." It was simply unacceptable for the daughter of a prominent doctor and civic leader to marry an oil field worker, as she put it. At the wedding and for at least the year that followed, Nettie was so rude to Harold that he finally told Elizabeth he would no longer be going with them to Okmulgee. Elizabeth wrote her mother and told her that none of them would be visiting and why, whereupon

Blossom went into action. Now my grandmother was one of the gentlest people I have ever known, but when she got her dander up, she was a force with which to be reckoned. And nothing could get her dander up more than keeping her grandchildren from her. So Blossom had a "talk" with her mother, and Nettie promised to "behave." In fact, Nettie eventually grew to love Harold, and they were close to each other, until her death in 1939.

And so the Hunsakers resumed their trips to Okmulgee for visits that were enjoyed by everyone. But the two who may have enjoyed those visits the most were Blossom and her granddaughter Frances Ann. Although the two women differed in age by more than sixty years, there was an enduring bond between them. Our grandmother took a nap every afternoon, and when she got up she would always have a cup of coffee. "It was the best coffee I have ever tasted," Francie (as we now call her) recalled some seventy years later. "I think it was because Okmulgee had great water." In any case, the young Francie Ann loved to join her grandmother for afternoon coffee, which for her was "coffee milk."

Most of all, Francie loved to hear her grandmother tell stories of when she was a little girl. A dreamy look would come into the older woman's eyes as she remembered those days. "One December, a few weeks before Christmas," Blossom recalled, "I saw a set of doll furniture in a store window. The chairs had velvet seats and, of course, nothing was plastic in those days. I went by the store everyday to admire the exquisite pieces, but I didn't dare tell anyone how much I loved them, because they were so expensive. Then, just a few days before Christmas, I went by and the set was gone...and I felt like crying. But on Christmas morning they were under our tree for me! It is one of my happiest childhood memories." Francie Ann would smile to think of her grandmother at the same age as herself on a Christmas morning and how happy she must have been. Blossom saved one of those miniature chairs over the years and showed it to her granddaughter when she was a teenager.

At another of their coffee times, Grandmother told Francie Ann what a healthy imagination she had as a child and how she loved playing "make-believe" with her friends: "One time we were playing 'getting ready for Thanksgiving' in the cold Nebraska fall. We crumbled leaves for vegetables and used rocks for potatoes but decided that a real potato would be perfect for the turkey. When we went in to ask mother for a potato, she saw our terribly red noses and blue fingers and said we must put on our gloves. 'Oh no, we're not cold!' we insisted. We were having so much fun and were afraid we would have to come in if we admitted we were cold." Whenever our grandmother would tell a humorous story like that, she would laugh in the most lady-like fashion with her mouth closed and her fingertips over her lips. It was a trait that Francie Ann cherished, as did we all.

Francie also recalls special moments with our grandfather. He worked long, hard hours and would come home for lunch and then take a short nap before going back to his office. On one occasion, he had to run an errand and little Francie Ann went with him. He parked the car in front of Ben Franklin, a small five-and-dime store. That disappointed Francie Ann, because she much preferred the larger Kress store.

"Grandpa," she asked, "why aren't we going to Kress? It's much bigger and nicer."

As they walked into Ben Franklin, her grandfather explained in a pleasant, conversational manner without any suggestion of lecturing. "Ben Franklin is owned by a person who lives in Okmulgee and all his profits stay in Okmulgee and Oklahoma. Kress is owned by a corporation from another state and the majority of their profits leave our state. You should support your locally owned businesses."

It was one of many valuable lessons that we learned from our grandfather.

Francie Ann's younger brother Hal also loved the family's visits to Okmulgee and especially enjoyed outings with our grandfather. Hanging on a wall in the old family barn were a number of bamboo fishing poles, and Hal loved nothing more than when they would take the poles down, drive out into the country, and spend the afternoon fishing.

I was fortunate to spend the first four years of my life in Okmulgee with my mother, grandparents, and Aunt Frances. Of course, what memories I have of that time are mostly from stories that I was told in later life. One of them had to do with my aunt. The old barn, where grandpa once kept his horse, had long since been converted to a garage for the family Buick. As you can imagine, the door was not particularly easy to manage. One day, I was with Aunt Frances when she needed to take the Buick on an errand and the door was not being cooperative.

"I can't get this damn door open," she exclaimed in exasperation. "Brucie, go get your grandpa and tell him we need his help."

I promptly ran into the house to relay my aunt's message. Unfortunately, not being familiar with the connotation of certain words, I relayed the message a bit too verbatim. To the best of my knowledge, no one had ever heard a curse word come from my grandfather's mouth. So you can imagine his dismay when he heard his young grandson relay his daughter's message.

"Grandpa, Aunt Francie can't get the damn door open."

I don't know exactly what transpired next, but I can only imagine the conversation that my grandfather had with his daughter.

In the waning months of 1945, my father came home from the war, and we moved to his hometown of Enid, where he set up his dental practice with his father. My life in Okmulgee had been pretty good. The truth is that I was undoubtedly spoiled by my mother, grandmother, and aunt. All that changed when we moved to Enid, since my father was a stern disciplinarian. But life picked up when my mother announced one day that I would soon have a little playmate in the house. And, sure enough, on December 11, 1946, my parents added to the list of grandchildren with the birth of my sister, Sally Sue. My first memory of her is when they brought her home and all the Shields family stood around the bassinet in our living room admiring the new arrival. I was intrigued when I overheard someone say, "She is the most beautiful baby in the world." Being at an age when children still take everything literally and believe they are the center of the universe, the comment was both interesting and logical to me. I remember looking down at her face for the first time and thinking, "So that's what the most beautiful baby in the world looks like." Having satisfied that curiosity, I went back to playing with my toys.

Our house was across the street from the elementary school, and I recall standing in our front yard, watching the big kids come and go, and looking forward to the day when I would be one of them. Of course, when that day finally arrived, I immediately began looking forward to the day when school would let out for summer break. And the main reason for that was that, right after school let out, my mother, Sally, and I would take the train for two glorious weeks with our grandparents in Okmulgee.

Uncle Charlie would meet us at the Tulsa train station and drive the thirty miles through five little towns to where our grandparents would be waiting for us. Although the family home and neighborhood had deteriorated considerably, it was still the nearest thing to heaven that I could imagine. Uncle Sam was still a bachelor and living at home, but he had moved into Elizabeth's old bedroom, which was quite a bit larger than the bedroom in which he had grown up. He had converted his old room into a ham radio layout, a hobby that he would pursue for the remainder of his life. Uncle Charlie lived in the smaller house next door. I also have fond memories of that house, with its smell of cigar smoke, where I would build model planes on Uncle Charlie's dining room table.

I was very fond of both of my uncles. Uncle Sam had a wonderful sense of humor, which I greatly appreciated, and Uncle Charlie was good-natured and fun. He loved his car, and I would occasionally go for a ride with him, the highlight of which was stopping at a country filling station to get a cold drink out of the ice-water container. Uncle Charlie was a great help to his sister Blossom, whom he still called Sally, and I can remember him covered in perspiration each night as he would wash the dishes for her.

Although having the fire station just across the drive from our grandparents' house might have been considered a negative by most people, it was definitely a positive for me. That is because the fire chief, whose family lived in an upstairs apartment in the station, had a son about my age. His name was Dude James. We became good friends and spent hours together playing in the fire station, where we were allowed to slide down one of the poles. Our favorite place, however, was Grandpa's barn. An old wooden ladder took us up to a loft that was simply utopia for young boys. There was a work bench and some tools in the loft, and we would spend hours building things like rubber band-propelled boats that we would sail in the fishpond beside the fire station or at a nearby lake.

Once I received a toy printing set, with rubber letters and numbers, an ink pad, and some paper. So Dude and I decided to go into the sign printing business. We found an empty basement space in downtown Okmulgee, with steps that led down to it from the sidewalk. There we set up our "business," with our first sign that announced we were open. Of course, no one came. Until noon that is, when my grandfather arrived and, in a very businesslike way, said he would like to purchase a "No Trespassing" sign for one of his country properties. And that was the extent of our business. It lasted one day but left a lifetime memory of my grandfather's love.

One of the benefits of life in Okmulgee was the chance to go downtown by myself. And one of my favorite places was the old Creek Council House, which had a museum section of local memorabilia. What drew me to it the most was that a picture of my grandfather hung on a wall in that room. It made me realize how important he was to the community, and I felt a great sense of pride.

My favorite room in our grandparent's home, with the possible exception of the dining room, was the sleeping porch. There was no air conditioning, and summers could be pretty hot even in early June. The sleeping porch was the coolest place, and I was usually allowed to sleep in one of the beds there. The sheets had a slightly musty smell from having been in place through winter and spring, and that aroma has always been associated with a sense of comfort for me. The only other thing I remember about the sleeping porch is that there were shelves filled with jigsaw puzzles, which was one of my grandmother's favorite pastimes.

I always felt a bit dejected to return to Enid. The highlight of my year was over. But one summer my father had a wonderful surprise waiting for us. While we had been gone, he built a toy train with an engine powered by a lawnmower motor and a red caboose that could seat two children. Not long after that, we moved to a new house several blocks from the old one, and I got to drive the train to it with some household goods in the caboose. That new house would be the one in which Sally and I would grow up, and before long there would be three of us children.

I was approaching the age of eleven when our mother announced to the family (somewhat to the surprise of my father, I think) that a new member of the family would be arriving in the spring. And so, on

March 22, 1952, Sally and I were thrilled to have a little brother. He was named Charles Robert and called Chuck. Now our grandparents in Okmulgee had seven grandchildren. Four more would be added when Uncle Sam later married, but our grandfather would not live to see that.

It was the time when the polio epidemic had everyone in fear. Our father made us stay in the house on hot summer days but did allow us to make our annual trips to Okmulgee. Like doctors across the country, the two Drs. Leslie struggled to manage their polio patients. I know that our grandfather worried about his grandchildren developing polio and did all he could to keep us safe during our visits. In 1955, he gave a great sigh of relief when he read that the FDA had approved the Salk vaccine. He would not live to witness the eradication of polio that the vaccinations would bring, but he knew that this was a major step toward that goal.

In the early 1950s, Grandfather Leslie broke down and bought a television, which he placed in the living room. Although he had been reluctant to make such an extravagant purchase, he soon joined the rest of us in its enjoyment. He liked to watch the news, especially in 1954 when it was announced that Eisenhower had defeated Stevenson for the presidency. His favorite TV programs were the westerns, like *Hopalong Cassidy* and *The Lone Ranger*. He was less enthusiastic about the introduction of rock and roll, which essentially began in 1954 with the likes of Bill Haley and the Comets and Elvis. Grandpa didn't think too much of that music but did see promise in the new *Disneyland* TV show, which debuted that same year on ABC.

I remember many pleasant evenings, sitting with the family and watching television in the living room of our grandparents' home. There were also some humorous moments that I recall. Uncle Sam had a dog named Bosco. He was a sweet dog but had one problem: flatulence. We would all be sitting in the living room watching a TV show, with Bosco lying on the floor beside Uncle Sam's chair, when the room would suddenly be filled with a most distinct odor. We kids would make a big deal of it, as though we were being gassed to death, which irritated Uncle Sam. He would get up and take poor Bosco outside, while the rest of us tried to suppress our laughter.

One of Grandpa Leslie's favorite pastimes was going for drives in the country, and he especially loved to have all his family go with him. The land around Okmulgee County is truly beautiful, and today I understand why he enjoyed the drives so much. As a young boy, however, all I really wanted to do was play, and those drives in the country took me away from that. So most of the time I hoped that I wouldn't be compelled to join the family on Grandpa's country drives. And yet, I now look back on the times when I did join the family on country drives with the fondest memories. I remember the tree-lined roads, and the dam and spillway, and Okmulgee Lake. I remember my grandfather singing and chatting and laughing when our grandmother would admonish him to keep his eyes on the road. And I would give anything if I could take one of those drives with them today.

Occasionally, on those country drives, we would stop at one of our grandfather's farms to visit with the tenants. That was not particularly exciting for us kids, except in the summer when the watermelons were ripe. One of Grandpa's many skills, which I truly admired, was his ability to take a large watermelon and crack it in half by hitting it on the edge of the farmer's front porch. He would then break it into smaller chunks and pass it around for all of us to enjoy. It is simple memories like that, of life with our grandparents, which never seem to fade.

Since our families were spread out across the state, the seven grandchildren didn't get together as often as we would have liked. When we did, however, we created happy memories of those times together. Hal and I are one year apart in age and especially enjoyed playing together. We were both a bit rambunctious, however, and prone to get into trouble. Francie Ann, on the other hand, seemed to be perfect and never got in trouble, and I guess that made me think of her as a bit prissy. As I grew older, however, I learned to appreciate her sweet nature, and she soon became one of my favorite people. I suspect we all have fond memories of those times together in our youth, but undoubtedly the one that will always stand out the most was our family reunion at Woolaroc.

The Woolaroc Museum and Wildlife Preserve is located near Bartlesville, Oklahoma, about forty-five miles from Tulsa. It was originally the 3,700-acre ranch of oilman Frank Phillips, later converted into a museum with Western art and artifacts, American Indian material, and one of the largest collections of Colt firearms in the world. In the fall of 1954, it was the venue for a Leslie clan reunion. The grandchildren ranged in age from two and a half to eighteen, with Chuck being the youngest and Tom Ed the oldest. We all enjoyed being together and learning a bit about the history of our state (well, at least the adults did, and the grandkids enjoyed playing together). Undoubtedly, the two who enjoyed it the most were Bruce and Blossom, who were surrounded by all their grandchildren and their families. Little could we have known then, however, that it would be the last time we would all be together with our grandfather. And that makes the occasion all the more meaningful and something that we still look back on with the fondest memories and the utmost thankfulness.

CHAPTER 14

Grovania

I
F BRUCE LESLIE HAD NOT BEEN A PHYSICIAN, the odds are pretty good that he would have been a pastor. Of all the hats he wore in his lifetime—healer of the sick, leader in his local and state medical profession, civic volunteer and philanthropist in his community, advocate of social justice, landowner, and astute businessman—the characteristic that most defined him was devotion to his faith. Maybe it began as a young boy in Arkansas, when his dying father gave him their family Bible. Maybe it was those solitary rides through Indian Territory, selling fruit trees, and the nights alone when he realized he was never alone. Maybe it was just the occasional breeze, swirling around his head, that caused him to look up and feel the presence of his Creator. Whatever it was, it began to manifest itself during his time in Denver, when he taught a young ladies' Sunday School class in his church and served as editor of the church's newsletter. It continued to reveal itself when he moved to Okmulgee and became active in his Methodist church, first teaching a Sunday School class and then becoming superintendent of all the church's Sunday School classes. But where it manifested itself the most, and what may be his greatest legacy, was when he resurrected a small country church called Grovania.

A few miles north of Okmulgee, on a corner of land bordered by two dirt roads, there was once a grove of fruit trees. Rumor has it that a young tree salesman had come through the area—back when it was called Indian Territory—in the late nineteenth century. In any case, old man Lewis, who owned a considerable amount of land, purchased a couple dozen trees and planted an orchard. The grove prospered and, as the world entered the twentieth century, the trees were bearing fruit and providing Mr. Lewis a tidy profit. By the early 1920s, however, disease and age were taking their toll on the trees, and Lewis began to consider alternative uses for that little corner of his property.

He had a friend of some entrepreneurial repute by the name of Frederick, and the two men began to hatch a plan to capitalize on the land where the declining grove of fruit trees still stood. The country was entering the Roaring Twenties, and people were looking for places to enjoy and celebrate life. In addition, prohibition had gone into effect in January of 1920, which meant that such places should ideally be in discreet locations away from suspecting eyes. A lonely corner of land, several miles outside of town, was just the ticket.

And so the grove of fruit trees came down and a two-room, white frame building was erected on the site. In order to give it an air of respectability, it was labeled as a community center. But they still needed a name for their building. After some consideration, Lewis and Frederick selected a name that commemorated the prior life of the little plot of land—they called it Grovania.

Throughout the Twenties, Grovania Community Center prospered. It hosted a variety of civic events during the week for the citizens of Okmulgee and the farmers in the surrounding area. But it was on Saturday nights that it truly came alive. Both town and country folk came for the dancing and socializing. The music could be heard for miles around. And in time it attracted the attention of law enforcement agents. A policeman would occasionally show up at the door of the center and would be met be Lewis or Frederick, who would assure the officer that there were no alcoholic beverages on the premises. A brief look around always confirmed the claim, and the good reputation of the Grovania Center remained intact for the duration of the Twenties.

But then, in October of 1929, the U.S. financial markets suffered a major crash. Over the next two years, markets around the world performed like roller coasters, until 1932 when they all collapsed with a devastating thud as the world entered the Great Depression. Both Lewis and Frederick suffered substantial reversals of their fortunes, and their community center was no longer in demand. People simply did not have the discretionary funds for entertainment. And so the lights eventually went out in Grovania, and the windows were boarded up.

Entertainment venues, of course, were not the only institutions to be afflicted by the Depression. Everyone felt the pain—including churches. When people are struggling to put food on their tables and keep a roof over their heads, charitable organizations are among the first casualties. And the smaller churches are usually the first to be hit. One of those was a small Baptist church on the outskirts of Okmulgee. Among its parishioners was Amos McIntosh Jr., whose father once ran the general store in downtown Okmulgee. Amos and his wife, Hettie, were loyal members of the church and did all they could to keep it afloat, but it was a losing cause.

As the collection in the plate became progressively smaller each Sunday, the time finally came when the little church could no longer support its pastor, and one day he sadly informed the congregation that he had accepted an assistant position in a larger church. A few of his flock went with him, and those who remained did their best to keep their church alive. But they could not even afford to pay the utility bills and the mortgage, and the building eventually reverted to the bank. On the last Sunday, there were only two families in the sanctuary: Amos and Hettie and their neighbors, the Herschel Simpson family, who owned a farm near them. They read some scripture and prayed and then discussed their options. They could, of course, join another church, but what appealed more to them—at least on a trial basis—was to begin meeting in one of their homes.

And so, on the following Sunday, the two families met in the McIntosh home for worship. They sang some hymns, read the Bible, prayed, and shared a few thoughts about their faith. Then they had lunch together.

It is well known that word can spread rapidly in a small community. By Monday afternoon, it was common knowledge that the McIntosh and Simpson families had started a "home church." Several of their friends, who weren't especially comfortable in a larger church, asked if they could join, and the following Sunday there were four families at the McIntosh home. Each family brought food, and they enjoyed a meal together after their service. One of them pointed out that this was how the early Christian church actually began: meeting in homes and sharing meals.

It wasn't long before the "flock" had become too large for the McIntosh home or any other home in the group. Something had to be done. One day, as Amos was driving down a dirt road toward Okmulgee, he noticed an old white-frame building that was boarded-up and obviously unoccupied. He had driven by it many times, but never thought much about it until that day. He pulled his pickup off the road and onto the grassy area in front of the building. Stepping up on the stone stoop, he saw a notice attached to the front door informing him that it had been the Grovania Community Center, and a phone number was provided for further information.

He stepped back to take a more critical look at the little building. It was in want of some repair and badly needed a new coat of paint. But as Amos tried to see it in his imagination—freshly painted, with the windows un-boarded and polished, and a little steeple above the front door—he thought this could well be the answer to prayers. So he wrote down the phone number and drove on.

When he called, the person on the other end of the line was a Mr. Lewis. Amos explained his interest in the old community center, and the two agreed to meet at the building. Amos brought Herschel and two other members of their new church with him, and Lewis came with Mr. Frederick. The building consisted of two rooms. The larger would be sufficient for their sanctuary and the smaller for Sunday School. After the tour, the men all sat down on some wooden benches to talk business. Lewis and Frederick were both church-going men and liked the idea of their center becoming a church. They offered Amos and his companions a ninety-nine-year lease at a monthly rental of $10. That would be about one dollar per month for each family, which was doable. The men all shook hands, and the Grovania Community Center became Grovania: A Community Church.

Grovania flourished during the Depression. Families living in the surrounding countryside appreciated not having to drive into town on Sunday mornings. They also felt more comfortable knowing that their meager offering each Sunday would be sufficient to cover the overhead of their church. Of course, they lacked many of the amenities of the larger churches. They could not afford a full-time pastor, although they would occasionally have a visiting minister, who was happy to preach for a few dollars and a good meal. They did not have a choir or an organ, a piano, or any musical instrument, although they enjoyed singing together and were sometimes accompanied when one of them would bring a guitar or fiddle. What they did have was each other, and they were a happy, thriving congregation. Until the war came.

By 1939, war in Europe seemed inevitable. The United States declared its neutrality, but most people could read the handwriting on the wall. Factories began to ramp up production in anticipation of supporting the war effort, and young men began to volunteer for military service. All this meant that jobs were coming back, and the economy was improving, and the Depression was receding as it was replaced by an even greater threat.

For churches in America, this meant a resurgence. People once again had some discretionary income with which to support charitable institutions, and churches were the main beneficiary of that. People may have also begun to feel a greater need for the church as they faced another world war, with loved ones going off to fight. In any case, the pews and the coffers began to fill up once again. However, people also wanted more from their churches. They wanted full-time pastors, choirs, organs, and the like. The big churches could provide all this. But for small churches, like Grovania, it was still not possible.

Gradually, attendance at Grovania began to decline. One by one, the families announced with great reluctance—and often with tears—that they felt the need to be in a larger church that could provide what they seemed to need during these trying times. Finally, one Sunday, the only two families to show up were again those of Amos and Herschel. They sat in silence for awhile, undoubtedly remembering the other time when they had sat together in the little Baptist church, just before they had closed it for good. They were determined not to let that happen again, although the future was anything but certain.

❦

Bruce Leslie was tired. He had been up much of the night before on house calls and had spent the day seeing patients in his office. Now, at 8:45 on a fall evening in 1940, he sat on a hard wooden chair with the fellow board members of the Methodist Church of Okmulgee. He might well have elected to miss the meeting that evening had it not been for the fact that the topic to be discussed was so critical to the future of their church.

The history of the Methodist Church in America is one of divisions and reunions. It was organized in Baltimore in 1784 as the Methodist Episcopal Church. In 1830, the Methodist Protestant Church split off, and in 1845, with the issue of slavery rocking the nation, the Methodist Episcopal Church, South, was established. Movements to reunite these factions began as early as 1870, but it was not until 1939 that the Methodist Church was created by the reunion of the Methodist Episcopal Church, the Methodist Protestant Church, and the Methodist Episcopal Church, South.

Not surprisingly, the question of reunion was highly controversial and led to heated discussions around the country during the 1930s, and the Okmulgee church was no exception. However, that was not the issue being discussed among the board members of the Methodist Church of Okmulgee that evening. The reunion had already occurred, and Dr. Leslie had been one of its ardent proponents. The question on the table that evening was, now that they were part of a nationwide denomination, whether it was time to have a new building for their church.

Most of the church members appeared to favor building a new facility at a new location. But one opposing view was that of Dr. Leslie. He felt that the expense of the construction and the move at this time would represent fiduciary malfeasance. Furthermore, he felt that the money could be better spent to help the marginalized in their community and beyond. Even though he was in the minority on the issue, Bruce felt that others would listen to his reasoning. After all, he had been a leading figure in the church for nearly forty years.

He had taught in their Sunday School, was currently superintendent of all the Sunday School classes, and had served on virtually every committee. He was clearly respected in their church. And that is why he had come to the Board meeting that evening—to make his case. He had prepared some remarks and, when it came his turn, he cleared his throat and began:

"As most of you know, the building we are in now was constructed in 1910. Not that long ago. It is still sturdy and adequate for the current size of our congregation. To take out a loan for new construction at this time, when the future of the economy is still uncertain, would create the risk of financial insecurity for our church. But, more important than that, there are so many people right here in our own community and around the world who are still desperate for our assistance. Wouldn't our money be better spent to help them? Isn't that what Jesus taught us?"

There was a long silence after Dr. Leslie had completed his remarks. Everyone looked down at the oak table in front of them, reluctant to make eye contact. There were a few more comments around the table, and then the chair of the Board called for the vote.

"All those in favor of building a new church please raise your hand."

Bruce continued looking down, with both hands on the table. When he slowly looked up, he saw that all other hands in the room were in the air, except for one elderly gentleman.

"All opposed."

Two hands were raised.

"The ayes have it."

Bruce looked around the room, making eye contact with each board member. He smiled at them and nodded as though to say he understood. But in his heart there was a painful feeling of emptiness.

Walking home that evening, he decided to stop by his office. He needed some quiet, solitary time to process what had just happened. He eased into the captain's chair beside his desk and sat in the darkness. For the first time since joining the church, he wondered if he belonged. He felt no animosity for anyone. These were his friends. But he wondered if they needed him anymore. It seemed that the world was moving on, and that he was no longer a part of it. He wondered what God had in mind for him. As he had done so often in times of doubt, he closed his eyes and fervently prayed for guidance.

The following morning, he returned to his office and checked the list of patients he was scheduled to see that day. One of them was young Amos McIntosh. His father had been one of the first people Bruce met when he moved to Okmulgee, and he had watched their son grow up to be a good farmer and a fine man. Amos had recently had an accident while working in the field, and Dr. Leslie wanted to make sure he was healing properly.

"So let's see how well you can move that arm," the doctor said when Amos was positioned on the examination table. He was pleased with his patient's range of motion and announced that the young man was once again "fit as a fiddle." Then the two men sat in the chairs by the desk and, as Bruce did with many of his patients, they chatted for awhile.

"How is it going with your country church?" the doctor asked.

Amos shook his head with a sad expression. "Not well I'm afraid, Dr. Leslie. People are going back to the bigger churches, and I fear we may have to shut down."

The two men sat quietly for several minutes, as Bruce began to ponder the irony of Amos coming in with this message just after last night's church meeting and his prayer for guidance. Was it simply a coincidence, or was he being gently guided? Well, there was only one way to find out.

"Would you mind if I joined you in worship this Sunday?" the doctor inquired.

The question shocked Amos. One of the most prominent citizens of Okmulgee coming to their little church! He couldn't imagine why he would want to do that, but he didn't want to seem rude.

"Why, of course sir," he blurted out. "We would be honored."

And so it was that Bruce Leslie drove out into the country in the fall of 1940 to attend worship service at Grovania Community Church. Amos and Herschel and their families were the only other ones there, and they had done their best to put together a respectable service.

Bruce did not interfere, but simply followed along with the songs, scripture, and prayer that they had prepared. In his mind, however, he couldn't help contrasting this moment with the formal service that he knew would be taking place at the Methodist Church. There was a simplicity and sincerity that touched him deeply. Much to his surprise, he felt a sense of belonging.

They invited him to have dinner with them, but Bruce said that Mrs. Leslie would have dinner on the table and that he had better get home. He did say, however, that he would like to come again next Sunday, much to the delight of Amos and Herschel. As he drove home that Sunday noon, his mind was awash with conflicting thoughts. Could he abandon the church that had meant so much to him over the decades? Did they still need him? Or could he be of greater service at Grovania? He obviously had to do some serious thinking—and praying.

After Sunday dinner, Bruce and Blossom sat together in their living room for a serious discussion. She knew that he had attended service at the little country church and assumed it would be a one-time visit. But she was surprised when he told her how it had affected him and that he was considering devoting his efforts to helping the church.

"So you would give up your position as a pillar of one of the largest churches in town to go out to a small, country church that may not even survive," she posited.

Bruce chuckled. His wife certainly had a way of boiling the facts down to their essence. "I guess that's pretty much the size of it," he responded with a smile.

Blossom smiled back and shook her head as though to say, "This is just like you." She knew better than to try to talk him out of anything he had set his mind to, and he assured her that he was still just testing whether this was right for him.

The following Sunday, there was another couple at the Grovania service. It was a fellow named Tom and his fiancé, Emily. They were both patients of Dr. Leslie and had been delighted (and amazed) when they learned that he was attending the country church. At the end of the service, they all stood in a circle and held hands to pray, and

Bruce felt a strange sensation pulsing through his body—a feeling as though he was receiving a message.

Before they left that day, Amos got up his nerve to ask the doctor a question.

"Dr. Leslie, we understand that you have been a Sunday School teacher for a long time, and we were wondering if you might give us one of your lessons next Sunday."

Bruce looked at Amos with a thoughtful, serious expression, although he was smiling on the inside. It felt like the message he had sensed was getting a little clearer.

"I would be honored," he responded, now letting the smile show through.

When he drove up onto the grassy parking area in front of Grovania the next Sunday morning, he was surprised to find that five other vehicles—three pickups and two cars—were already there. Inside the church, he was greeted by a sizable group of people, both adults and children. He shook hands with each of them, and it is hard to say who was happiest—the people or the doctor.

After everyone was seated on the wooden benches, Amos led them in some hymns. They had a few old hymnals, entitled *Songs of Faith*, which contained most of Bruce's favorites. Each family had brought their own Bible, and these were used next for the reading of scripture. Herschel then led them in prayer before introducing Dr. Leslie, who he announced would "bring the word." The doctor made it very clear that he was not a preacher and that this would not be a sermon, but rather a Bible lesson, which he hoped would not bore the children, who giggled at being acknowledged.

Bruce Leslie opened his Bible to the book of Matthew and read from the eighteenth chapter: "For where two or three are gathered in my name, there I am in the midst of them."

"Looking around at each of you this morning," he began, "I have no doubt that this word is being fulfilled in our midst today, just as it was for the first Christians. They must have been greatly comforted by this assurance from Jesus. We know from the Pentecostal story in Acts that it was the Holy Spirit which came to them when they were together after the resurrection and which guided them as they sought to do God's will. And I believe that our church, which is the people of Grovania, have the same desire to please God and the same Spirit to guide us."

He went on to describe how the early Christian church began as small groups in homes or caves or any safe place they could find, and how they helped each other by looking out for those in need, and how they shared meals together, and how they grew in God's grace. And he compared that to the congregation of Grovania and predicted that, with the guidance of the Holy Spirit, they could do the same.

There were a few tears in the room that morning as the doctor concluded his remarks, and then they each came up to him with handshakes and hugs. They told him how much they hoped he would stay with them. They said they needed him. It touched him deeply, but at some point Bruce Leslie had already decided that this is where God meant for him to be.

At the next meeting of the Methodist Board, Bruce tendered his resignation as superintendent of their Sunday School classes. He explained that he felt a calling to do what he could for the people of Grovania Community Church. He told them how much he would miss each of them and that he intended to retain his membership in the Methodist Church of Okmulgee and to keep in touch and join them as often as possible. And he assured them that he would continue to support the church, including making a major gift to the capital campaign for the construction of their new building.

And so the decade of the Forties passed. The war came to an end, and the young men and women came home and started new lives. And through it all, Grovania flourished under the leadership of Dr. Bruce Leslie. He not only taught from the Bible every Sunday morning—which his congregation thought was as good as any sermon—but he also organized the services, leading the singing and selecting the scripture passages that were appropriate for that week's lesson. As a young boy in the late Forties and early Fifties, I have fond memories of going to Grovania with my grandparents when we would visit them in Okmulgee. My most vivid memory is of my grandfather standing before the little congregation leading them in the hymns. After his death, I was fortunate to receive his personal hymnal, in which he had marked some of his favorite hymns: "The Lily of the Valley," "There is Power in the Blood," and "Shall We Gather At the River."

Blossom did not accompany her husband to Grovania on most Sundays during the Forties, but toward the end of the decade she announced to Bruce one morning that she was going with him. It surprised and amused him and brought back a memory of long ago when she had announced, as a young wife, that she would be going with him on a nighttime house call in the country. Of course, he was delighted to have her join him at Grovania, and it turned out to be the beginning of a partnership in the church, with Blossom organizing the Sunday School classes for the children and helping with the congregational meals after many of the services.

By the dawn of the Fifties, the faithful of Grovania had become like family to both Bruce and Blossom. And their little flock felt the same way about them. For a decade, Dr. Leslie had sung with them, read scripture with them, and worshipped with them. Many of them were his patients, and he had helped bring several of them into the world. Tom and Emily were married now and had a newborn named Luke. When the little guy was just old enough to say a few words, he became fascinated by the church bell in the steeple. One Sunday, he expressed his interest.

"Me pull!"

Everyone laughed, and Dr. Leslie bent down, picked up Luke, and let him pull the rope to ring the bell. From that day on, it was the doctor and his "helper" who rang the bell every Sunday morning to call the faithful to worship. And there was another custom that caused Luke and all the children to gather around the doctor when they first arrived at Grovania each Sunday. He always carried candy in his pocket, and all the children would hold out their hand to receive their treat.

Amos and Hettie McIntosh had remained pillars of the little church and not only attended faithfully but were always there to help in any way they could—mowing what little grass there was, making repairs to the building, and helping Blossom with Sunday School class for the children and meals for the congregation. Their son, Ben, was now a teenager and passionate about all sports. He seemed prone to injury, however, and Dr. Leslie was frequently having to patch him up.

With the exception of the McIntoshes, who had some Creek blood, the makeup of the congregation was all white, and a day came when their Christian charity would be challenged. It was a time when racial hatred was again in the news. One day, Bruce's old friend Jeremiah came to his office for a routine checkup. His health had forced him to close his barber shop, and he had recently lost his wife. Many of his friends had also died and he no longer felt comfortable in his church. Jeremiah was lonely. As the two men sat and talked, the doctor wondered how he would be accepted at Grovania.

"Well, Jeremiah," he began slowly. "I have found a small group of kindred spirits in a little country church who have given me great comfort. Maybe you would find a place for yourself there also."

"Ah 'preciates that, Doctuh, but does you reckon them white folks would accept a colored like me?"

Bruce was quiet and pensive for awhile. The same question was bothering him, and he wasn't sure of the answer. Finally, he looked up at Jeremiah and said, "I'll ask."

The following Sunday, his Bible lesson was on the inclusivity of Jesus—how he accepted all people. In fact, it seemed that the more marginalized they were, the more he wanted to reach out to them. Some of the people in the congregation that morning may have connected the dots, when the doctor told them that there would be a brief business meeting after the service. When he told them that he wished to propose a new member and who it was, there was deafening silence as everyone looked down at their knees. Finally, Herschel slowly stood up.

"Doctor Leslie," he began hesitantly, "any friend of yours is good enough for me." Then his voice became more forceful. "And I ask anyone who feels the same way to stand with me."

Again, it was quiet, and no one moved for what seemed like a long time. Then Amos stood up beside his friend, and Hettie and Ben joined him. Tom and Emily followed, and soon everyone in the room was standing. At that point, Bruce was choking back his emotions and finally spoke.

"Let us pray."

The following Sunday, Bruce and Blossom brought Jeremiah with them. It was awkward at first. Everyone tried to be welcoming, but probably tried too hard. As the weeks and months passed, however, it became more natural, until the time came when everyone seemed comfortable with everyone else. In fact, they soon came to love Jeremiah as much as Bruce had for decades. And that was the way it went at Grovania as the years passed by. It was a small band of simple folks who loved the Lord and loved each other. And their leader, Bruce Leslie, never failed to thank God for guiding him to this place in his life.

In 1955, Bruce celebrated his eighty-first birthday. He and Blossom seemed to be enjoying good health, and he still went to his office everyday, although the number of patients he saw had diminished over recent years. He no longer took night calls. He was happy to leave that to the young doctors like Sam and his partner. They still lived in the old house on East Third, and Sam still lived there with them, having yet to find the right person to be his wife. Charlie, who was by now a confirmed bachelor, still lived in the smaller house next door. Everyone seemed to be content with their lives, and their joy was always made greater when a set of the grandchildren and their parents would come for a visit.

One area in which Bruce Leslie had not slowed down was his leadership at Grovania. In fact, he spent more time than ever preparing his lessons. One Saturday morning, as the leaves were beginning to fall, he sat at his desk and tried to consolidate a theme that had been on his mind. He was thinking about the Old Testament story of the Israelites, who, after forty years of wandering in the desert, stood at the Jordan River but were afraid to cross over. He thought he might title the lesson, "Crossing the Jordan."

That evening, he sat alone with Blossom and told her the general outline of his lesson for the next morning. She looked at him with a sense of foreboding and felt a chill go through her, but then let it pass and said she thought it sounded good.

And so, on a crisp autumn morning, Bruce and Blossom Leslie sat beside each other in their Buick and headed for one more time down a dirt road toward the little country church called Grovania.

Epilogue

LOSSOM LESLIE lived for nearly two more decades after the loss of her husband in 1955. She passed peacefully on June 26, 1974, in the home that Bruce had built and to which he had brought his young bride in 1909. The family had encouraged her to move to more modern accommodations, since both the house and neighborhood were continuing to deteriorate. But like her husband, she was not willing to move. Maybe it was the memories that caused her to stay—memories of the house that she and Bruce made into a home, where their children grew up, and where their grandchildren loved to come for visits.

Her brother Charlie never married. He continued to live in the smaller house next door until after Dr. Leslie's death. Then he moved into the main house so that he could be closer to his sister and take care of her. A downstairs bedroom was added, so Blossom would not have to negotiate the stairs so often. After her death, Uncle Charlie was all alone in the big house. He passed away the following year.

Blossom lived to see the fourth and final marriage of her children. In 1963, Sam Leslie married Dolores Dahl. She had two children by her previous marriage, John Bruce and Elizabeth Suzanne, who were ten and nine years old, respectively, at the time of their mother's second marriage. The Leslies added two more to their family, Samuel Brewster III in 1963 and Dianna Dahl in 1966. Sam changed his medical specialty to ophthalmology, and the family moved to Oklahoma City and then to Albuquerque, New Mexico, where he ran the eye clinic at the Veterans Administration Hospital.

The four Leslie children, Elizabeth, Frances, Ruth, and Sam, and their spouses all lived full and blessed lives. Most of them lived to see the final decade of the twentieth century or the early years of the twenty-first. In all, they gave their parents, Bruce and Blossom, eleven grandchildren, twenty-seven great-grandchildren, thirty-five great-great-grandchildren (at last count), and six great-great-great-grandchildren. (See family tree: The Family of Samuel Brewster and Blossom McKeage Leslie.)

All the grandchildren are still living (as of this writing) except for three. Tom Ed Echols and his wife, Judy, had three children before he was killed flying helicopters for a petroleum company in the 1960s. Judy remarried and moved with her children to Italy. No further information is available on her family. Suzanne Leslie Kupferer died August 20, 2020, and Sam Echols died June 16, 2021. The family has also lost two great-grandsons—Harold Robert (Robbie) Hunsaker on January 1, 2020, and John Robert Shields on December 5, 2020— and one great-great-grandson, Austin Brook Harkey on December 3, 2006.

The family home our grandfather built, and the houses adjacent to it, are all gone now. In their place is simply a grassy vacant lot. In 2012, my sister, Sally Autin, and I returned to Okmulgee to revisit the site and to relive some of the memories associated with it. All that remains today is the brick wall that once surrounded the main house and the concrete steps that led up to it. The fire station is still there, but the upper level, where Dude James and his family once lived, has been removed. The small brick building that was Gilstrap's grocery store, across the street from the Leslie home, is still there, although boarded up and long since vacated.

Downtown Okmulgee hasn't changed a great deal. The stone Creek Council House still occupies the center green and now houses a museum of Creek Nation history and a gallery of Native American art. Our grandfather's picture, which once hung in the building, is no longer there. I was told that it is most likely in a warehouse along with hundreds of other artifacts that have passed through that stone structure over its history of more than a century. Just off the town square, on East Main Street, the building still stands where Dr. Bruce

Leslie practiced medicine for his entire career. It was closed the day we visited, but I stood on the tile steps that led up to it and thought of how many thousands of times his feet must have passed that way.

Sally and I drove north of Okmulgee to where the little church called Grovania once stood. It too is gone. In its place is a larger metal building that is occupied by a congregation of Free Will Baptists and is called Grovania Free Will Baptist Church. We had arranged to meet one of the deacons of the church, and he gave us a tour of their facilities. I must confess that it is much nicer and more up to date than the previous two-room wood-frame church that once stood on that same piece of ground. But for Sally and me, there was a bit of sadness that an important part of our childhood was gone. Our spirits were lifted somewhat, however, as we prepared to leave and saw a painting near the front entrance—a lovely rendition of the first Grovania. (See photos.)

The fact that the family home and the original Grovania are no longer there is actually comforting in a way. Both would undoubtedly be in considerable disrepair by now, and it is far better to have the memories of those former times, when the Leslie homestead rang with the laughter of a loving family, and the little wood-frame church was filled with singing and worship as the faithful were led by Dr. Bruce Leslie.

Only a few of his grandchildren were alive or old enough at the time of his death to have known or remembered our grandfather, Dr. Samuel Brewster Leslie Sr. And even those of us who were old enough to remember were too young at the time to appreciate what a remarkable life he had lived and what a wide range of contributions he made to his community and to all those whose lives he touched. Without family support, he educated himself and became a successful physician and a leading citizen of his community. During his lifetime, he was there when Oklahoma achieved statehood, he lived through two world wars and the Great Depression, and he witnessed the introduction of cars, aviation, radio, television, and much more. He was not only a pioneer doctor in Okmulgee, but a local and statewide leader of his medical profession, a longtime proponent and leader of his town's education programs, a champion of social justice, a landowner and accomplished businessman, and a pillar of the Methodist Church of Okmulgee and of Grovania Community Church.

His descendants continue to benefit to this day from our grandfather's astute business acumen. In the final weeks of his life, after his heart attack, his son, Sam, was amazed that his father could recall from memory the details of each of his land holdings. This was vitally important to him, because he knew it would be the source of ongoing financial support for Blossom and their progeny. Today, his grandchildren and their families continue to receive payments from the mineral rights of the land he began to acquire nearly a century ago.

But, of course, his legacy is far more important to his family than just being beneficiaries of his financial success. He left us with a sturdy model for living. He taught us to not only respect all people, but to have compassion for them, especially the downtrodden, and to do whatever is in our power to make life better for others. He taught us to respect this planet we live on and to appreciate the beauty of our world and to care for it. He taught us to laugh and to sing and to make the most of each day that we are given. And, most importantly, he taught us to remember the source of all our blessings and to never fail to show our profound gratitude for all that we have.

As is true of so many American families, we descendants of Bruce and Blossom Leslie are blessed to have been born into a family that not only provided the opportunity for prosperity and success but taught us the values of a meaningful and grateful life. And, if our grandfather was with us today, he surely would remind us that our blessings go back over the ages—through the generations of our family who put their faith in God. He would remind us of the faith of the first Leslie—old Bartoff—in ancient Scotland and how that faith sustained generations of Leslies as they traveled over the seas to Ireland and then to the New World. He would recall for us the trials they faced as they journeyed through the Carolinas, Kentucky, Tennessee, Arkansas, and Indian Territory that would become Oklahoma. He would remind us of the wars and the illnesses they endured and the challenges of working the land and moving on in search of a better life. And he would surely want us to remember that, through all these challenges, it was faith in their Creator that sustained each generation of our heritage. What greater legacy can one generation leave to another?

And, just maybe, Dr. Leslie would also recall for us those times that he felt a gentle breeze swirl about his head, as his ancestors before him may have also experienced, causing them to look up and to sense the presence of the Spirit in the wind, assuring them, and us, of God's ever-abiding love.

Family Tree

Children*	Grandchildren	Great-Grandchildren

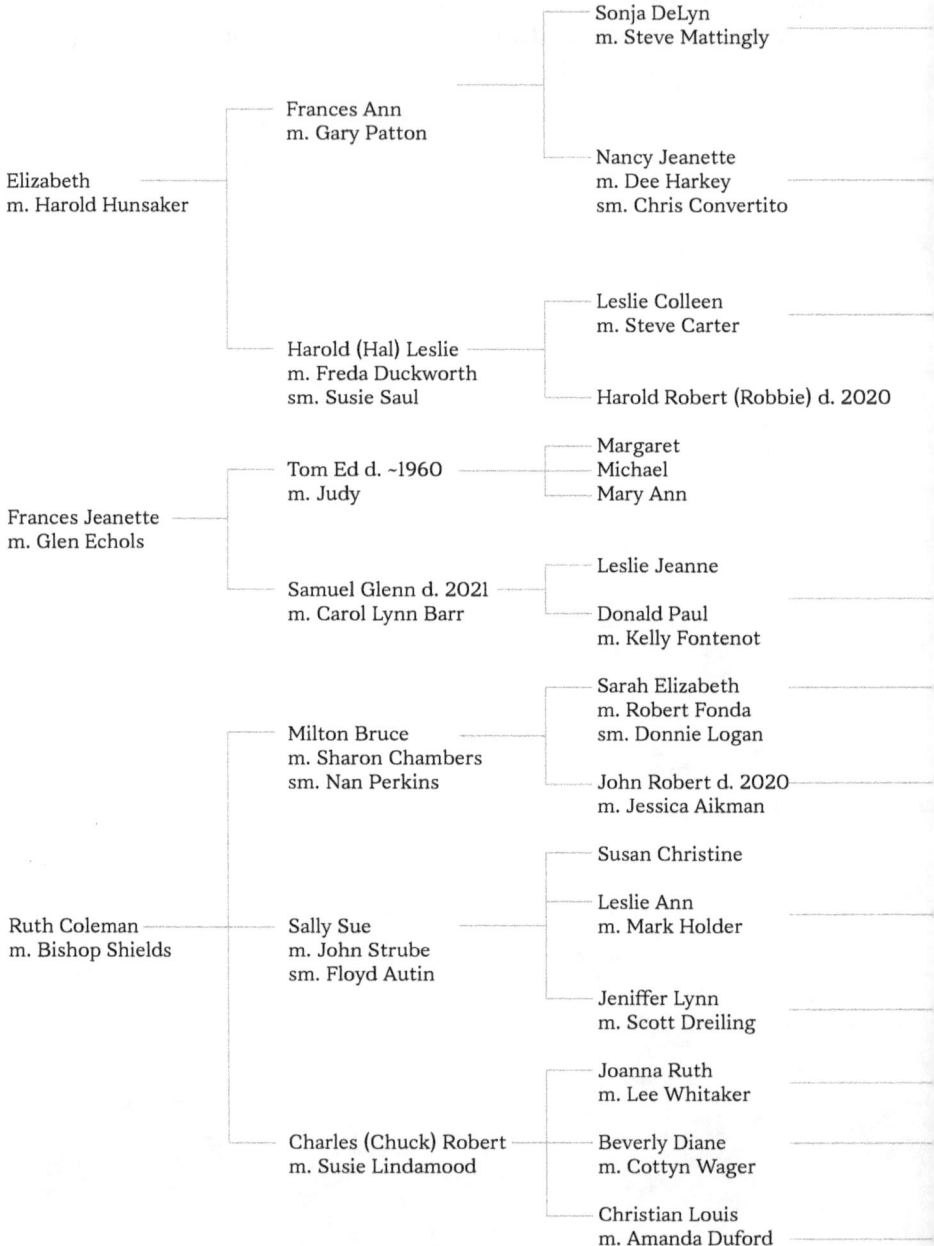

Elizabeth
m. Harold Hunsaker

- **Frances Ann**
  m. Gary Patton
  - Sonja DeLyn
    m. Steve Mattingly
  - Nancy Jeanette
    m. Dee Harkey
    sm. Chris Convertito
- **Harold (Hal) Leslie**
  m. Freda Duckworth
  sm. Susie Saul
  - Leslie Colleen
    m. Steve Carter
  - Harold Robert (Robbie) d. 2020

Frances Jeanette
m. Glen Echols

- **Tom Ed d. ~1960**
  m. Judy
  - Margaret
  - Michael
  - Mary Ann
- **Samuel Glenn d. 2021**
  m. Carol Lynn Barr
  - Leslie Jeanne
  - Donald Paul
    m. Kelly Fontenot

Ruth Coleman
m. Bishop Shields

- **Milton Bruce**
  m. Sharon Chambers
  sm. Nan Perkins
  - Sarah Elizabeth
    m. Robert Fonda
    sm. Donnie Logan
  - John Robert d. 2020
    m. Jessica Aikman
- **Sally Sue**
  m. John Strube
  sm. Floyd Autin
  - Susan Christine
  - Leslie Ann
    m. Mark Holder
  - Jeniffer Lynn
    m. Scott Dreiling
- **Charles (Chuck) Robert**
  m. Susie Lindamood
  - Joanna Ruth
    m. Lee Whitaker
  - Beverly Diane
    m. Cottyn Wager
  - Christian Louis
    m. Amanda Duford

The Family of Samuel Brewster & Blossom McKeage Leslie

Grt. Grt. Grands

Grt. Grt. Grt. Grands

Molly Frances
m. Alex Breitenbach

Romy Alice
Fiona Frances

Caroline Coleman
m. Jake Marshall

Reid Patton

Austin Brook d. 2006

Elizabeth (Libby) Leslie
m. Aaron Goedde

Ellie Louise
Mason Parker
Rhett Austin

Madelyn Belle
e. Michael Ryan Stanley

Claire Elizabeth

Jackson Paul

Samantha Katherine

Allison Leah Fonda
e. Hunter Logan

Nathan Edward

Anna Ruth
Lila Mae

Nathan Scott
Grace Ruth

Addison Ruth
Jillian Zane

Carsyn Robert

Ezra Charles
Hannah Sharon
Esther Sue

Key:

*	all deceased
d.	deceased
m.	married
sm.	second marriage
e.	engaged

Continues next page

Children*	Grandchildren	Great-Grandchildren
Samuel Brewster Jr. m. Dolores Dahl	John Bruce m. Sharon Swift sm. Carolyn Engel	Brian Christopher m. Anna Leavengood
		Steven Stewart m. Jessica Soares
	Elizabeth Suzanne d. 2020 m. Bill Webster sm. Carl Kupferer	Amy Webster m. Todd Hinnerichs
		Burke Webster m. Stephanie Ackerman
		Whitney Kupferer m. Jamie Barnhart
		Zak Kupferer
	Samuel Brewster III m. Carrie Troester	Aaron Joshua
	Dianna Dahl m. Richard Pool sm. Charles Morey	Travis James Pool m. Tanja Schwartz
		Tanner Leslie Pool e. Mary Nguyen
		Trevor Richard Pool m. Madison Anders

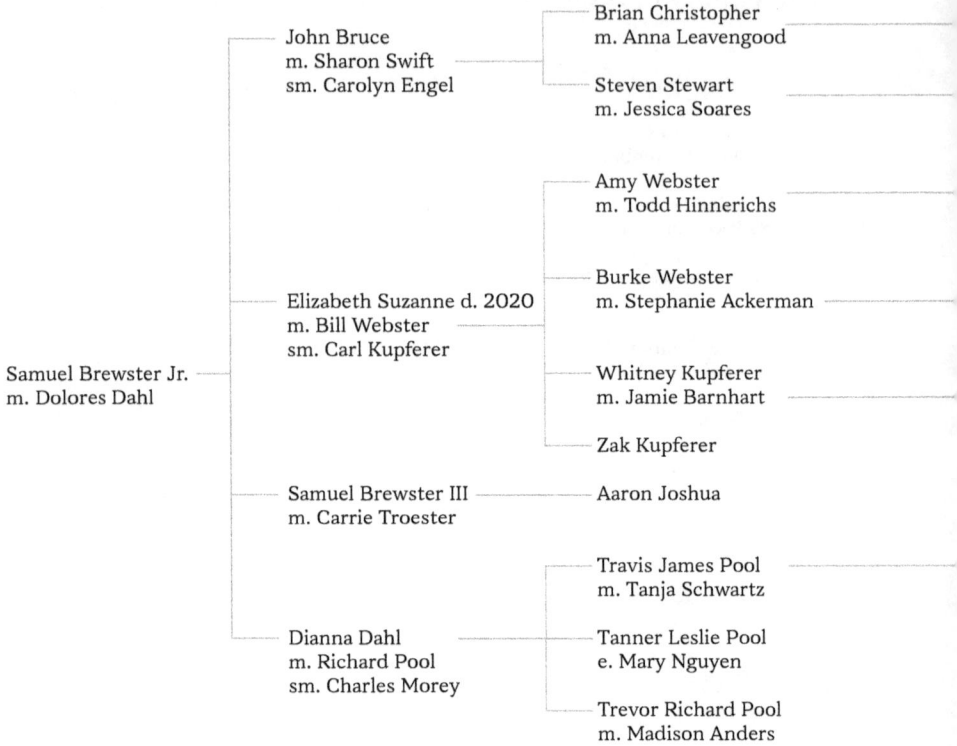

Grt. Grt. Grandchildren

Roan David
Liam Bruce

Alistair Kellan
Brennan Myles

Reese Katherine
Taylor Newton
Tristin Noah
Sadie Dahl

Walker Samuel
Owen Burke
Gemma Roxann

Savannah Brooke
James Brady
Kinsley Reese

Jameson Kenneth

Key:

*	all deceased
d.	deceased
m.	married
sm.	second marriage
e.	engaged

Acknowledgements

THE WRITING OF THIS BOOK has been a family effort, with generous contributions from most of the living adult descendants of Bruce and Blossom Leslie. But there are two people for whom I am especially indebted for their invaluable assistance: my cousin Frances Ann Patton, and my wife, Nan Phipps Perkins.

Francie wrote a brief history several years ago of our grandmother, Blossom Eliza McKeage Leslie, which is both touching and full of helpful information. She also organized an "oral history" conversation among the three Leslie sisters in their later years and then transcribed it, providing more priceless records for our family archives. In addition to these two documents, which provided many stories for the book, she graciously assisted me with research and further information throughout the decade of writing the book.

Nan and I lost our spouses of 50 years at about the same time and were married in 2018. She spent most of her career at Elon University, where she served as vice-president of both admissions and development. As an English major, her writing skills were highly valued at Elon and are a Godsend for me. She was essentially my editor and best critic of the book, carefully reading each chapter for grammatical improvement as well as suggesting structural changes to clarify passages and improve the flow of the book. My sincere thanks to both Francie and Nan.

I am also grateful to many others members of our family for their assistance with documents, pictures, and additional information: my sister, Sally Autin; my brother, Chuck Shields; and my cousins Hal

Hunsaker, Delyn Mattingly, Leslie Echols, Don Echols, John Leslie, Samuel and Carrie Leslie, and Dianna Morey.

In 2012, I made a research trip through Arkansas and Oklahoma to gather information for this book and encountered many generous and helpful people along the way. Before leaving on the trip, I spoke by phone with Bennie Davis, the city manager of Leslie, Arkansas, and he recommended that I contact and visit Herschel Simmons, a great source of local knowledge. Mr. Simmons, who was ninety-three years old at the time, graciously invited me into his home and could not have been more helpful. In addition, his sister Becky and son Mark joined us. Becky had driven over to nearby Marshall to make copies of some pages on the Leslie family from a local history book in the library, and Mark drove me around town in his pickup, pointing out sites of interest and introducing me to some of Leslie's citizens, including Mr. Davis. My deepest gratitude to each of them.

Larry Hoffman runs an auto repair shop adjacent to the Leslie Cemetery, and he gave me a book with names of those buried in the cemetery, which was very helpful during the hour or so I walked around looking for family markers. Mr. Hoffman also recommended that I contact Joe Bratton, who is also a great-great-grandson of Samuel Leslie. Joe and I had a delightful chat on his front porch and concluded that we are distant relatives. He writes a local column for the Marshall newspaper (Leslie no longer has a paper) and was a wealth of information.

I had planned to spend my last day in Leslie at the Ozark Heritage Center. But, to my great disappointment, it was closed, and I was about to leave, when the curator, Jeff Stansbury, stepped out of the building. I explained my situation, and Mr. Stansbury graciously spent the next two hours giving me a personal tour of the museum, which had a great deal of information on the town and my family, including a picture of my great-great-grandfather. (See photos.)

Before leaving Leslie, I stopped by a gift shop called Elk and Eagle and had a nice chat with the proprietor, Darryl Treat, who provided more information about the history of the area, as well as some memorabilia. I am deeply grateful to all the generous and helpful people I met in Leslie, Arkansas.

I had also made advance arrangements to meet someone at the Grovania Free Will Baptist Church, near Okmulgee, Oklahoma, where the original Grovania once stood. My sister Sally and I were met there by Deacon Glenn Bohuslavicky, who let us in and gave us a tour of the church. I am grateful to him and to church clerk Bonita Fredericks for the historical background of Grovania that is the basis for the story in Chapter 14.

There is one more person to whom I owe a debt of gratitude, although we never met. Marion Emerson Murphy was a retired vice admiral of the U.S. Navy, who spent years of his retirement researching the Leslie family and recording it in a book titled *Early Leslies in York County, South Carolina; Their Migrations to Tennessee, Missouri and Arkansas; Their Ancestry and Descendants*. Although our family lines diverged at some point, he traced the Leslie lineage from the ancient Scots up to the 1970s, including my family. His efforts are the framework upon which the early history of the Leslie clan in this book is based.

I also wish to thank Ms. Linda L. Roghaar and all her excellent team at White River Press for transforming my raw manuscript into this handsome volume.

References

Allen, Arthur. *Vaccine: The Controversial Story of Medicine's Greatest Lifesaver*, W. W. Norton, 2007.

Barry, John M. *The Great Influenza; The Story of the Deadliest Pandemic in History*. New York: Penguin Books, 2018.

Brands, H. W. *Andrew Jackson; His Life and Times*. New York: Doubleday, 2005.

Burke, Bob. *Miracle at Guthrie: The Founding of Oklahoma*. Oklahoma Heritage Association, 2011.

Dary, David. *Frontier Medicine: From the Atlantic to the Pacific 1492–1941*. New York: Alfred A. Knopf, 2008.

Ehle, John. *Trail of Tears: The Rise and Fall of the Cherokee Nation*. New York: Anchor Books, 1988.

Haller, John S. *The History of American Homeopathy: The Academic Years, 1820–1935*. London: Pharmaceutical Products Press, 2005.

Leslie, Blossom. *Life of S. B. Leslie, M.D.* (unpublished).

Luckerson, Victor. *Remembering Tulsa: 100 Years Later; The Promise of Oklahoma; How the Push for Statehood Led a Beacon of Racial Progress to Oppression and Violence. Smithsonian*, April 2021, pp. 26–35.

Ludmerer, Kenneth M. *Time to Heal: American Medical Education from the Turn of the Century to the Era of Managed Care*. Oxford: Oxford University Press, 1999.

Kieffer, Beth. *Images of Okmulgee*. Mt. Pleasant, S.C.: Acadia Press, 2016.

Maclean, Sir Fitzroy. *Scotland; A Concise History*, 4th edition. New York: Thames & Hudson, 2012.

Madigan, Tim. *Remembering Tulsa: 100 Years Later; Confronting the Murderous Attack on the Most Prosperous Black Community in the Nation. Smithsonian*, April 2021, pp. 36–51.

Magnusson, Magnus. *Scotland; The Story of a Nation*. New York: Grove Press, 2000.

McCourt, Malachy. *History of Ireland*. New York: MJF Books, 2004.

McIntosh, Billie Jane. *From Georgia Tragedy to Oklahoma Frontier: A Biography of Scots Creek Indian Chief Chilly McIntosh*. American History Imprints, 2008.

Murphy, Marion Emerson. *Early Leslies in York County, South Carolina; Their Migrations to Tennessee, Missouri and Arkansas; Their Ancestry and Descendants*. 1972 (privately printed).

Patton, Frances Hunsaker. *Blossom Eliza McKeage Leslie* (unpublished). onthisday.com

Robins, Natalie. *Copeland's Cure: Homeopathy and the War Between Conventional and Alternative Medicine*. New York: Alfred A. Knopf, 2005.

Steele, Phillip W. and Steve Cottrell. *Civil War in the Ozarks*, Revised Edition. Gretna, LA: Pelican Publishing Company, 2009.

Woolery, D. R. *The Grand Old Lady of the Ozarks*, Fifth Edition. Hominy, OK: Eagles Nest Press, 2005.

About the Author

BRUCE SHIELDS is a retired ophthalmologist who spent his career in academic medicine as a professor at Duke University and professor and chairman at Yale University. His previous publications are primarily scientific, with books, chapters, and journal articles focused on his chosen field of glaucoma. His *Textbook of Glaucoma* is currently in its seventh edition. His only prior non-scientific book is entitled *Gifts of Sight*, released in 2012, which recounts experiences with patients at Duke and Yale who taught him lessons in life through the way they approached their medical challenges. He lost his first wife, Sharon, in 2015 and subsequently married Nan Perkins, who is a retired vice-president of Elon University. Bruce and Nan live happily in their home in Burlington, North Carolina.

www.ingramcontent.com/pod-product-compliance
Lightning Source LLC
Chambersburg PA
CBHW021759190326
41518CB00007B/367